# drink
## to your health

# drink
## to your health

### Anita Hirsch, M.S., R.D.

**Delicious, Easy-to-Prepare**

**Juices, Smoothies,**

**Teas, Soups,**

**and Other Beverages**

**That Deliver**

**Vitality and**

**Immunity**

**marlowe and company**
**new york**

Published by
Marlowe & Company
841 Broadway, 4th Floor
New York, NY 10003

DRINK TO YOUR HEALTH: *Delicious, Easy-to-Prepare Juices, Smoothies, Teas, Soups, and Other Beverages That Deliver Vitality and Immunity*

Library of Congress Cataloging-in-Publication Data
Hirsch, Anita, M.S.
        Drink to your health : delicious, easy-to-prepare juices,
    smoothies, teas, soups, and other beverages that deliver vitality and
    immunity / by Anita Hirsch.
            p.  cm.
        ISBN 1-56924-651-3
        1. Beverages—Therapeutic use.  2. Tonics (Medicinal
    preparations)  I. Title.

    RM239 .H57 2000
    615'.321—dc21
                                                                990-42187

9  8  7  6  5  4  3

DESIGNED BY PAULINE NEUWIRTH, NEUWIRTH & ASSOCIATES, INC.

Printed in the United States of America

Distributed by Publishers Group West

This book is dedicated with thanks to my mom, Mildred Sher, who taught me to eat with health in mind, to cook with love for those you love, to recycle leftovers, and be delighted with a fresh peach for dessert.

# Contents

## 4  cocktails and other sparkling beverages

## 5 soups, broths, and hot beverages 123

## 6 milks 149

## 7 staples

## ailments index

Thank you to my always-patient husband, Sy, who suggested the title, and who tasted and critiqued all of my experiments. (I told Sy to expect a beverage for every meal including breakfast. He said "I've tasted my first glass of toast.") Thank you to my daughter Leanne, who called whenever she found something that I should include, and to my son, Michael, who kept me abreast of the latest food trends.

Thank you to my colleague, Jane Zeigler M.S., R.D., C.N.S.D., assistant professor and director for the Allen Center For Nutrition at Cedar Crest College in Allentown, Pennsylvania, who reviewed my manuscript. Thank you to Deborah Gore, R.D., who guided me down realistic and practical nutritional paths. Thank you to Marian Wolbers and Brenda Bortz, who lovingly shared their creativity and energy. Thanks both to my agent Ellen Greene and to my editor Matthew Lore. Thanks also to Pauine Neuwirth for a terrific book design, Susi Oberhelman for a beautiful cover, and Eileen DeWald for marshalling the manuscript through production.

A huge thank you to Diana Delling, the editor who whipped the manuscript into shape.

ESHA Research, Inc., The Food Processor, was used to analyze the recipes for nutrition content.

# Introduction

You may have heard that tea helps prevent heart disease and cancer. You may have heard that cranberry juice can prevent or cure urinary tract infections. You may have even heard that soy milk fights cancer and may help ease the symptoms of menopause.

Well, all of these things are true. And as you'll learn by reading and using this book, beverages can deliver many other powerful health benefits—and taste great, too.

The beverages in this book promote vitality and immunity. Some of them will lift your spirits when you're down in the dumps, while some will help your body fight off a cold or flu. Some of these drinks will energize you, some will help you relax after a long day on the job. If you suffer from a chronic illness, you'll find something in this book that may help you achieve optimal health. And if you're worried about getting enough vitamins and minerals in your daily diet, there's a drink in this book that can help you, too.

## the choice is yours

After twenty-eight years in the food and nutrition field (twenty-two of them spent developing and testing recipes for health books and magazines), I have some strong opinions about a healthy diet. You need to choose foods that will benefit your health. Don't pick foods simply because you are hungry for them, because they will fill you up, or because they are convenient. And don't eat strawberry shortcake when plain strawberries will do.

Unfortunately, when it comes to beverages, Americans seem to be making choices that are quick and convenient rather than sound and healthful. Milk consumption is down, while soft drink consumption continues to rise. Sugars and other sweeteners, coming mostly from soft drinks, currently account for 20 percent of the calories in the average American teenager's diet. In 1994, the average teenager drank 64.5 gallons of soft drinks each year, up from 20.6 gallons in 1978!

Many of the popular new bottled coffee and tea drinks are brimming with sugar. If you check the labels carefully, you'll see that one bottle of sweetened iced tea contains 2.5 servings, or more than 200 calories, and provides hardly any vitamins or minerals.

Even the "juice" drinks we buy for our children (and for ourselves) are suspect. Too often they are little more than water, high fructose corn syrup, artificial flavors and colorings, and preservatives. Most contain less than 2 percent real juice!

But there *are* alternatives. A fresh fruit drink prepared from a recipe in this book (Mango Milk, for example) may cost about $1 per serving—a little more than a commercial juice drink, perhaps, but you're getting so much more nutrition for your money. The delicious fresh fruit drinks and smoothies in this book are naturally sweet and colorful (your kids will love them). They provide our bodies with important vitamins, dietary fiber, and lots of healing phytochemicals. And they *don't* contain high-fructose corn syrup.

## quick meals for those on the go

In these fast-paced times, it can be hard to find time for a full sit-down meal. A healthy beverage, carried in a mug or thermos, makes a wonderful, nutritious meal on the go.

Beverages should not substitute for every meal; sitting down to eat a meal with others can be healing in itself. But a healthy drink is certainly a better choice than a vending-machine selection or a greasy fast-food meal. Nutrient-dense drinks—those that provide lots of nutrients for every calorie they contain—make excellent meal replacements. (Try the Morning Superstart when you don't have time for breakfast.) Even the soups I've included in this book can be puréed and sipped on the road.

## make beverages part of your healthy diet

Juice drinks, smoothies, and puréed soup beverages are great ways to add fruits and vegetables to your daily diet. The National Cancer Society recommends at least five servings a day of fruits and vegetables for optimum health; I've heard other experts advocate up to 10 servings of fruits and vegetables a day, including one high-vitamin C fruit or vegetable at every meal.

Healthy beverages are also delicious ways to provide your body with vitamins, minerals, and nutrients you wouldn't otherwise be getting in your daily diet. A cup of tasty Doubly Green tea provides a hefty dose of immune-strengthening vitamin C, for example. And one serving of the Hi-Po smoothie supplies almost half the day's requirement of potassium.

Each recipe in this book is followed by a nutrition analysis that provides information on the calories, protein, carbohydrates, fat, cholesterol, dietary fiber, and sodium contained in each serving. Most of the recipes are low in fat (less than 5 grams per serving), low in sodium (less than 300mg), and high in dietary fiber (3g or more). If you wish to reduce your intake of refined sugar, feel free to substitute a non-caloric sweetener when sugar is called for.

The analysis also notes which vitamins and minerals are abundant in each drink. Drinks labeled "high in" a nutrient contain at least 20 percent of the recommended Daily Value of that nutrient. Drinks labeled "a good source of" a nutrient contain between 10 and 20 percent of the recommended

Daily Value of that nutrient. Look for beverages with flavors that appeal, the nutrients you need, or both!

## medicinal drinks

Do you have a specific health problem or concern? There may be a beverage that can help prevent that disease or provide relief from your symptoms. Herbal teas have medicinal properties—echinacea tea, for example, can strengthen the immune system and help shorten the duration of a cold. And certain foods contain nutrients that make them beneficial for persons with specific medical conditions. Foods that are rich in calcium, magnesium, and potassium, for example, can actually help control high blood pressure. For information on which beverages are recommended to treat or prevent specific health conditions, consult the Ailments Index on p.189.

## don't forget the water

I encourage you to try as many of the recipes in this book as you can. But I also urge you to remember the most important healthy beverage of all: water. Our need for water is second only to our need for oxygen. Water makes up more than half of our body weight and is a necessary component of all our vital body fluids: blood, the digestive juices, urine, and perspiration. Water plays a crucial role in every one of our bodily functions and transports nutrients throughout our bodies.

Drink at least 8 glasses of clear, fresh water—2 quarts— a day. Carry it with you in a bottle or thermos, or keep it in the refrigerator at home and at work. Leave a water bottle or glass in full view on your desk; it will serve as a reminder to drink more water.

## drink to your health

*Drink to Your Health* is filled with more than 125 delicious, fast, and easy to prepare beverages. These drinks are made using healthful ingredients that are available in your local supermarket or health food store. They are naturally sweet or require minimal amounts of added sweeteners. And none of them rely on artificial flavors or colors for their great taste.

A stove or microwave and an immersion or regular blender or a food processor are all the equipment you'll need to prepare the beverages in this book. (Sometimes little more than a long-handled iced-tea spoon or a simple hand-held whisk will do.) An electric juicer is required in a few of the recipes, but because juicing removes most of the dietary fiber from a fruit or vegetable, I've kept juicer-processed drinks to a minimum. Most of the juices and smoothies included here are made by puréeing fruits and vegetables in a blender, which preserves their valuable fiber content. To prepare these blender drinks or smoothies when on the go or at a tailgate party, you can purchase a blender that plugs into a vehicle's cigarette lighter.

I hope you find that these delicious drinks make an important contribution to your good health, and that *Drink to Your Health* becomes a trusted and important addition to your library of cookbooks.

# 1

Cool, refreshing juice drinks combine sweet fruit and vegetable juices to create beverages with exciting new flavors and optimal nutritional benefits. Generally high in vitamins A and C, juice drinks are excellent immune system strengtheners.

## juices
### plain and fancy

# Arthritis Relief

Fresh strawberry and pineapple juices make this refreshing drink high in vitamin C, an antioxidant thought to be particularly beneficial for those with rheumatoid arthritis. Vitamin C promotes collagen production and the repair of connective tissue. Those who take aspirin for pain relief should be sure to include extra vitamin C in their diets because aspirin depletes the body's natural supply.

> ½ cup fresh strawberry juice (8 to 10 strawberries)
> ½ cup fresh pineapple juice (about 3 cups pineapple chunks)
> ⅛ teaspoon sugar (optional)
> Ice

Combine the ingredients, add ice, and enjoy.

**yield:**
> 1 serving (1 cup)

**per serving:**
> 106 calories, 1 g protein, 26 g carbohydrates, 0.5 g total fat, 0 cholesterol, 0 g dietary fiber, 3 mg sodium. High in vitamin C. A good source of vitamin $B_6$, folate, and potassium.

# Cancer Phyter

Tangy, nutrient-packed Cancer Phyter is high in sulforaphane glucosinolate (sulforaphane GS), an antioxidant and phytochemical found in cruciferous vegetables that stimulates the body's immune system and may help reduce the risk of some types of cancer. It's made with BroccoSprouts, a nutritional broccoli sprout developed by the Johns Hopkins University Medical Center. A one-ounce serving (about ½ cup) of BroccoSprouts contains as much sulforaphane GS as 1½ cups of cooked broccoli—so a little of this drink goes a long way. Look for BroccoSprouts in your grocery store's produce department.

If BroccoSprouts aren't available, use fresh broccoli instead. You'll get a slightly sweeter beverage, but you'll need to drink more to get your dose of sulforaphane GS.

> ½ cup Brocco Sprouts, rinsed, or 1 stalk raw broccoli,
>    rinsed and trimmed
> ½ cup carrot juice (5 or 6 carrots)
> ½ clove garlic
> 1 teaspoon chopped onion

Combine the ingredients in the juicer and juice. For a less tangy taste, add more carrots. Serve.

**yield:**
   1 serving (½ cup if using sprouts; 1 cup if using broccoli)

**per ½ cup serving with sprouts (estimated):**
   38 calories, 2 g protein, 8 g carbohydrates, 0.2 g fat, 0 cholesterol, 0 dietary fiber, 62 mg sodium. High in vitamin A, vitamin C, and beta carotene.

# phytochemicals

Phytochemicals, or plant chemicals, are substances found in fruits and vegetables that scientists believe can prevent disease in humans and help us maintain healthy immune systems. Further research may shed light on just how and why phytochemicals work in our bodies. While some manufacturers are trying to isolate them in pill form, eating a variety of fruits and vegetables is the best way to make sure that phytochemicals are included in your diet.

| phytochemical | food |
| --- | --- |
| Allium | onions, garlic, scallions, leeks, chives |
| Caffeic acid | fruits |
| Carotenoids: | |
|     alpha and beta carotene | orange vegetables and fruits |
|     lutein | green leafy vegetables |
|     lycopene | tomatoes, red grapefruit, guava, watermelon |
|     cryptoxanthin | tangerines, papaya, oranges, mango, peaches, nectarines |
| Coumarins | citrus fruits, parsley, carrots |
| Dithiolthiones | cruciferous vegetables: kale, broccoli, cauliflower, Brussels sprouts, cabbage, bok choy, collards, mustard and turnip greens, rutabaga, turnips |
| Ellagic Acid | grapes, blueberries |
| Ferulic Acid | fruits |
| Flavonoids: | |
|     Quercetin | tea, wine, apples, onions, celery |
|     Kaempferol | cranberries, grapes, broccoli, endive |
| Indole-3 carbinol | Cruciferous vegetables |
| Isoflavones | |
|     Genistein | Soybeans, kidney beans, chickpeas, lentils |
| Isothiocyanates: | |
|     sulphorophane | Cruciferous vegetables |
| Lignans | Flaxseed |
| Limonene | Citrus fruits |
| Phytic Acid | Grains |
| Phytosterols | Soybeans and dried beans |
| Protease inhibitors | Soybeans and dried beans |
| Saponins | Soybeans and dried beans |

# Tutti Fruiti on the Rocks

Prune juice is the old stand-by when it comes to constipation relief, but not everyone likes its taste. This drink combines prune juice with apricot nectar to improve its flavor and add the benefits of vitamin C and beta carotene. Tutti Fruiti makes a good breakfast drink. Try one every morning to promote regularity.

> ½ cup apricot nectar
> ½ cup prune juice
> Ice

Combine and serve over ice.

**yield:**
1 serving (1 cup)

**per serving:**
161 calories, 1 g protein, 41 g carbohydrates, 0.2 g fat, 0 cholesterol, 2 g dietary fiber, 9 mg sodium. High in vitamin A (and beta carotene which is utilized as vitamin A). A good source of carbohydrates, vitamin B$_6$, vitamin C, iron, and potassium.

# Faux Café

Allentown, Pennsylvania, registered nurse Marie Melick finds that warm prune juice does the trick for her patients with constipation. Served with a touch of milk, a cup of Faux Café in the morning should bring relief.

½ cup prune juice
2 tablespoons 1 percent milk

Warm prune juice in a mug in the microwave or in a small pot on the stove. Add the milk and serve warm.

**yield:**
1 serving (½ cup)

**per serving:**
104 calories, 2 g protein, 24 g carbohydrates, 0.4 g fat, 1 mg cholesterol, 1 g dietary fiber, 21 mg sodium. A good source of vitamin B6 and potassium.

# High-C

A terrific boost for the body's immune system, High-C contains 73 mg of vitamin C—more than 100 percent of the recommended Daily Value. Tomatoes supply additional cancer- and disease-fighting nutrients.

> ½ cup chopped tomatoes
> ½ cup orange juice
> 1 teaspoon lemon juice
> 1 teaspoon honey

Combine ingredients in blender and process until smooth.

**yield:**
1 serving (1 cup)

**per serving:**
104 calories, 2 g protein, 23 g carbohydrate, 0.3 g fat, 0 cholesterol, 1.3 g dietary fiber, 32 mg sodium. High in vitamin C and folate. A good source of vitamin A, thiamine, iron, and potassium.

# choosing
## canned tomatoes

Tomatoes are loaded with vitamins A and C and contain the protective phytochemical lycopene. Flavorful, fresh, in-season tomatoes kept at room temperature (not refrigerated) always taste best. But canned tomatoes can be an excellent and convenient substitute. Choose a brand that's low in salt. Canned tomatoes can sometimes taste metallic or salty; those labeled "fresh cut" or "fresh flavor" are often good bets. I like Del Monte fresh cut, no-salt-added tomatoes, but do your own taste test and see what you like.

# Ginger Apricot Support

Support your good health! Apricots, both fresh and canned, are an excellent source of carotenoids, thought to prevent cancer, heart disease, and stroke. Use bottled apricot nectar or make your own apricot purée (purée fresh or canned, drained apricots in a blender). Yogurt with active cultures and ginger root give this drink even more nutritional appeal.

> ¼ cup plain nonfat yogurt
> ¼ cup spring water or mineral water
> ⅛ teaspoon grated ginger root
> ½ cup apricot purée or nectar

Combine ingredients in a glass and stir to blend.

**yield:**
1 serving (1 cup)

**per serving:**
105 calories, 4 g protein, 23 g carbohydrates, 0.2 g fat, 1 mg cholesterol, 1 g dietary fiber, 52 mg sodium. High in vitamin A. A good source of calcium.

# ginger

Fresh ginger, found in the produce sections of most grocery stores, can help calm an upset stomach, prevent motion sickness, and stimulate appetite. It's also good for relieving migraine headaches.

Choose a piece that is firm and without blue or moldy spots. To store, wrap and place the ginger in the produce drawer in the refrigerator, then use as needed. The skin can be removed or eaten for added fiber. You can juice fresh ginger by slicing it and running the slices through a garlic press. Or use a ginger grater, sold in Asian food markets.

# One-Two Punch

Start with this buttermilk-based beverage—buttermilk is a good source of calcium, which can help prevent osteoporosis. Then follow it up with a little sunshine; the vitamin D that your body makes from exposure to the sun will help deposit the calcium in your bones.

One-Two Punch is particularly recommended for those nursing broken bones. The vitamin C in the pineapple juice helps the body repair bones and generate collagen, which holds the bones together.

> ½ cup pineapple juice, fresh or canned
> ½ cup buttermilk (1 percent fat)
> 1 teaspoon granulated sugar or mint syrup
> (see page 178)
> mint leaf (for garnish)

Combine ingredients in a glass and serve. For extra froth, use blender to combine.

**yield:**
1 serving (1 cup)

**per serving:**
136 calories, 5 g protein, 27 g carbohydrates, 1 g fat, 4 mg cholesterol, 0.3 g dietary fiber, 130 mg sodium. High in vitamin C. A good source of calcium, riboflavin, and potassium.

# Elizabeth's Healing Cocktail

Elizabeth, who lives in New York City, stops for a healthy beverage every day on the way home from her high-powered job. Her favorite is this combination of raw vegetables—it's high in fiber, antioxidants, and protective phytochemicals.

The sweetness of the carrot and orange juices hide the bitterness of the cabbage juice. If you like, add more carrots to tame its strong flavor. In folk medicine, cabbage and cabbage juice are used to heal ulcers. In one recent study, ulcer patients who drank a quart of cabbage juice daily showed signs of improvement.

> ⅛ small head of cabbage
> 3 carrots
> 1 orange, peeled
> ¼ small clove garlic (optional)
> ¼ teaspoon fresh ginger (optional)

Combine ingredients in a juice machine. Juice and serve.

**yield:**
  1 serving (⅔ cup)

**per serving (estimated):**
  184 calories, 5 g protein, 44 g carbohydrates, 1 g fat, 0 cholesterol, 0g dietary fiber, 96 mg sodium. High in vitamin A, thiamine, niacin, vitamin B$_6$, vitamin C, folate, calcium, magnesium, potassium. A good source of protein, carbohydrates, riboflavin, vitamin E, pantothenic acid, iron.

# cruciferous
# vegetables

High-fiber cruciferous vegetables help ward off colon, rectal, and other cancers. Add them to soups, salads, and vegetable juice drinks whenever you can. The family of cruciferous vegetables includes:

Arugula

Bok choy

Broccoli

Brussels sprouts

Cabbage

Cauliflower

Collards

Kale

Kohlrabi

Mustard greens

Radishes

Rutabaga

Turnips and turnip greens

Watercress

# Piquant Pomegranate

Fresh pomegranates generally appear in the fall of the year. We used to buy them and eat them on the way to school. Mom would drop some seeds into a sandwich bag and we would suck the juice out of them. Mom knew what she was doing–pomegranate juice is high in vitamin C, so the snack provided an immune system boost just at the start of the cold and flu season. This drink will do the same.

> ½ cup fresh pomegranate juice
> 1 cup water
> 2 tablespoons frozen apple juice concentrate
> ½ teaspoon sugar or fructose or other sweetener

Combine the ingredients in a glass, stir, and serve.

**yield:**
1 serving (1½ cups)

**per serving:**
115 calories, 0.4 g protein, 29 g carbohydrates, 0 fat, 0 cholesterol, 0 dietary fiber, 10 mg sodium. A good source of vitamin C and potassium.

# juicing
## a pomegranate

You can juice a pomegranate in either a juicer or a blender. To juice in a blender, cut the pomegranate in half, scoop out the seeds and the surrounding pulp, and place them in the blender. Turn on the blender for a few seconds—the blender blades will separate out most of the juice. Add a small amount of water and blend for a few more seconds, then pour the juice and seed mixture into a strainer. The juice can be pressed out or strained into a glass. One pomegranate should yield about $\frac{1}{2}$ cup of juice.

# Good Time Party Punch

Keep party guests happy *and* healthy with this nutritious punch. Every serving packs 67% of the DV of vitamin C (40mg), so you can actually encourage them to overindulge. Pineapple juice is also high in potassium and folate (folic acid), which can help prevent heart disease. For extra kick, add fresh ginger juice (see page 17).

> 2 cups cranberry juice cocktail
> 2 cups pineapple juice
> ¾ cup ginger syrup (see page 176), 12 ounces
>     ginger ale (see p.24), or ¾ cup fresh ginger
>     juice (see p.17)

Combine and serve. For just one serving, use ⅓ cup of cranberry cocktail, ⅓ cup of pineapple juice and 2 tablespoons of ginger syrup, ginger ale, or fresh ginger juice.

**yield:**
  6 servings (about 1 cup each)

**per serving:**
  108 calories, 0.4 g protein, 27 g carbohydrate, 0 fat, 0 cholesterol, 0.3 g dietary fiber, 4 mg sodium. High in vitamin C.

# ginger ale

When choosing a commercial ginger ale, check the ingredients label. If it doesn't contain natural ginger, don't bother. Health food stores typically carry natural ginger ales—look for Health Valley brand or Reed's Original Ginger Brew and Raspberry Ginger Brew from the Original Beverage Corporation.

You can also make your own ginger ale using ginger syrup (see page 176). This flavorful syrup can be prepared and refrigerated to use for many drinks.

# 2

Prepared in a blender, smoothies combine frozen or fresh ripe fruits with healthful soy, rice, or dairy milks and yogurts. These thick, colorful drinks deliver phytochemicals and antioxidant vitamins along with protein and lots of flavor.

# smoothies
## and other blender drinks

# Nutrient-Dense
# Pear-Avocado Abundance

High in fiber and packed with nutrients, this extra-thick beverage makes a healthy snack or meal. Drink it all at once, or divide it up and drink portions throughout the day. With selenium and zinc, it's an excellent flu- and virus-fighter. And because it's high in calcium, magnesium, and potassium, it can also help keep blood pressure under control.

$\frac{1}{2}$ avocado, peeled and chunked
$\frac{1}{2}$ pear, peeled and chunked
$\frac{1}{2}$ cup plain fortified soy milk
$\frac{1}{4}$ cup plain nonfat yogurt
$\frac{1}{4}$ cup apple juice (more if you prefer a thinner drink)
2 teaspoons wheat germ

Combine all ingredients in blender and process until smooth.

**yield:**
1 serving ($1\frac{1}{2}$ cups)

**per serving:**
366 calories, 13 g protein, 47 g carbohydrates, 17 g fat, 3 g sat fat, 8 g mono fat, 1 mg cholesterol, 11 g dietary fiber, 109 mg sodium. High in protein, beta carotene, vitamin A, vitamin C, thiamine, riboflavin, vitamin $B_6$, vitamin $B_{12}$, vitamin E, folate, calcium, magnesium, copper, and potassium.

# Mango Sunrise

Mango Sunrise is high in antioxidants, making it another great choice for the immune system. Wheat germ adds selenium and zinc, which are often lacking in our diets, but you can skip the wheat germ if you'd prefer a smoother textured drink. If you're not an orange juice fan, try substituting cranberry juice or vitamin C-fortified apple juice.

> ½ mango, cubed
> ¼ cup orange juice
> ½ cup vanilla-flavored fortified soy milk
> 1 tablespoon toasted wheat germ (optional)
> Dash nutmeg

Combine the mango, orange juice, soy milk, and toasted wheat germ (optional) in a blender and process until smooth. Garnish with freshly ground nutmeg.

**yield:**
1 serving (1 cup)

**per serving without wheat germ:**
170 calories, 4 g protein, 36 g carbohydrates, 2 g fat, 0 cholesterol, 2 g dietary fiber, 48 mg sodium. High in vitamin A, vitamin $B_{12}$, vitamin C, vitamin E, folate. A good source of thiamine, niacin, vitamin $B_6$, vitamin D, pantothenic acid, calcium, magnesium, and potassium.

**per serving with wheat germ:**
197 calories, 6 g protein, 39 g carbohydrates, 3 g fat, 0 mg cholesterol, 3 g dietary fiber, 48 mg sodium. High in vitamin A, vitamin $B_{12}$, vitamin C, vitamin E, folate, thiamine, and magnesium. A good source of riboflavin, niacin, vitamin $B_6$, vitamin D, pantothenic acid, calcium, iron, potassium, selenium, and zinc.

# choosing
## a soy milk

Look for a soy milk that's fortified with extra vitamins and minerals. For soy-based drinks or smoothies, I recommend vanilla-flavored or plain fortified soy milks from Eden Foods and Imagine Foods. These brands are fortified with calcium and vitamin $B_{12}$, nutrients that are present in dairy milk but not in regular soy milks. Edensoy Extra and Soy Dream are also fortified with beta carotene, Vitamin E, and Vitamin D; one serving of either provides 4 percent of the recommended Daily Value for iron.

## on the  go

Canned soy drinks are not always easy to find, but they make great, convenient alternatives to soda when you need an easy, portable drink. Yeo's Soy Drink Deluxe, found in Asian markets, is a delicious plain soy drink made with soybean extract, water, and sugar. One can contains 210 calories and 31 grams of sugar, which is comparable to a soda, but also provides 8 grams of protein, 4 percent of the Daily Value of calcium, and 6 percent of the Daily Value of iron. Samantha's brand fruit soy drinks, found in health food stores, are also healthy choices.

# Melon Mango Invigorator

Melon Mango Invigorator makes an excellent snack. It's low in calories, a good source of protein, and brimming with vitamin C, vitamin A, and beta carotene. And because it's made with soy milk, it contains isoflavones that can help protect your body against cancer and heart disease. Taste this one before you add sugar—you may find that it's sweet enough just as it is.

½ mango, cubed
½ cup cubed cantaloupe
½ cup fortified soy milk
1½ teaspoons sugar

Combine ingredients in a blender and purée. Serve.

**yield:**
1 serving (1 cup)

**per serving:**
185 calories, 6 g protein, 37 g carbohydrates, 3 g fat, 0 cholesterol, 3 g dietary fiber, 62 mg sodium. High in vitamin A, vitamin C, folate, and B$_{12}$. A good source of protein, carbohydrate, dietary fiber, thiamine, niacin, vitamin B$_6$, vitamin D, calcium, magnesium, and potassium.

# Caribbean Powerhouse

Movie character Rocky Balboa gulped a beverage full of freshly cracked eggs before his runs through the streets of Philadelphia. Today we know that raw eggs can carry hidden bacteria, so this twenty-first century version of Rocky's power drink is made with a sterilized egg product.

$\frac{1}{2}$ cup skim milk or fortified soy milk
1 banana
$\frac{1}{4}$ cup unsweetened pineapple juice
$\frac{1}{4}$ cup egg substitute
$\frac{1}{2}$ teaspoon sugar
$\frac{1}{4}$ teaspoon vanilla extract

Combine ingredients in a blender and purée. Serve.

**yield:**
1 serving ($1\frac{1}{3}$ cup)

**per serving with skim milk:**
228 calories, 12 g protein, 45 g carbohydrates, 1 g fat, 2 mg cholesterol, 3 g dietary fiber, 165 mg sodium. High in protein, vitamin $B_6$, vitamin C, calcium, and potassium. A good source of carbohydrates, dietary fiber, vitamin A, riboflavin, vitamin D, folate, copper, magnesium, and phosphorus.

# Hi-Pro

**Try this drink** instead of using a high-protein powder. The egg substitute, milk, and peanut butter together deliver 19 grams of protein—more than a third of the day's requirement. The peanut butter also adds zinc, folate, and vitamin E. And Hi-Pro is high in calcium, magnesium, and potassium—three minerals that help keep blood pressure under control.

1 banana
½ cup skim milk
¼ cup pineapple juice
¼ cup egg substitute
2 tablespoons peanut butter
½ teaspoon sugar
¼ teaspoon vanilla extract

Combine all ingredients in a blender and process until smooth. Serve.

**yield:**
1 serving (almost 2 cups)

**per serving:**
414 calories, 19 g protein, 52 g carbohydrates, 17 g fat, 3 g sat fat, 2 mg cholesterol, 5 g dietary fiber, 167 mg sodium. High in protein, dietary fiber, riboflavin, niacin, vitamin $B_6$, vitamin C, folate, calcium, copper, magnesium, and potassium. A good source of vitamin A, thiamine, vitamin D, vitamin E, pantothenic acid, iron, and zinc.

# Orange Julia

Add a few simple ingredients to a glass of orange juice and you've made a good thing even better. Nutritional yeast adds selenium and lots of B vitamins; the protein in the powdered milk and egg white make this drink frothy, creamy, and delicious.

1 cup orange juice
1 teaspoon powdered nutritional yeast
3 to 4 teaspoons powdered skim milk
4 teaspoons powdered egg white
dash sugar (optional)

Combine ingredients in a blender and blend for about 30 seconds. Wait a few seconds for the egg white to absorb the liquid, then blend again for a few seconds. Serve.

**yield:**
1 serving (about $1\frac{1}{2}$ cups)

**per serving:**
169 calories, 12 g protein, 30 g carbohydrate, 1 g fat, 1 mg cholesterol, 1 g dietary fiber, 141 mg sodium. High in protein, thiamine, riboflavin, niacin, vitamin $B_6$, vitamin $B_{12}$, vitamin C, folate, pantothenic acid, and selenium. A good source of vitamin A, magnesium, and potassium.

# powdered egg white

Pasteurized powdered egg white is a safe, convenient alternative to fresh raw egg whites, which may contain salmonella bacteria. Look for Just Whites brand in the baking supplies section of your supermarket (near the condensed and evaporated milks) or order it by mail (see Resources). Two teaspoons of the product equals one egg white; an 8-ounce can contains the equivalent of more than 4 dozen whites. It can be stored on the shelf, and you'll never waste yolks again! Just Whites even makes a nice meringue when mixed with water.

# Mike's Blueberry Egg Cream

Egg cream, my son's favorite drink, contains neither egg nor cream. The popular New York beverage is traditionally made from chocolate syrup, milk, and seltzer. Here, blueberries replace the chocolate for a drink that's naturally sweet and low in calories. The anti-aging properties of blueberries can't be beat, and they help prevent urinary tract infections, too.

> ½ cup fresh or frozen blueberries
> ½ cup 1 percent or skim milk or soy milk
> ½ cup seltzer

Combine the blueberries and milk in a blender and purée. Pour into a glass and add the seltzer. Stir and serve.

**yield:**
> 1 serving (1 cup)

**per serving with 1% milk:**
> 92 calories, 5 g protein, 16 g carbohydrates, 2 g fat, 5 mg cholesterol, 2 g dietary fiber, 67 mg sodium. High in $B_{12}$, vitamin D, and calcium. A good source of riboflavin and vitamin C.

# the anti-aging
## power of berries

Blueberries and cranberries contain ellagic acid, a substance that helps to protect us from the free radicals which cause aging and contribute to or accelerate disease. Berries are also high in vitamin C, the free radical-fighting antioxidant that can help prevent aging and age-related illnesses such as heart disease, cancer, and even prevent cataracts.

Like blueberries, cranberries are high in ellagic acid, which slows aging and tumor growth. Cancer and heart disease can be hindered by cranberries, and cranberry juice has a reputation for fighting urinary tract infections. And the flavonoid quercetin helps prevent cancer and free radical damage.

# Soy Peach Blueberry Perk-Up

High in fiber, low in fat, and packed with the antioxidant beta carotene, vitamin E, and vitamin C, this drink can help prevent cancer and so much more. Soy protein (from the soy milk) is believed to prevent heart disease, while the combination of protein, magnesium, fiber, and vitamins makes it a good choice for those with chronic fatigue syndrome. The Perk-Up provides two full servings of fruit (remember, five a day) to boot. Cheers!

> ½ cup fortified soy milk
> ½ cup blueberries, fresh or frozen
> 1 peach, peeled and quartered or ½ cup frozen sliced peach
> 1 teaspoon lemon juice
> 1 teaspoon nutritional yeast

Combine ingredients in a blender and purée. Serve.

**yield:**
1 serving (about 1 cup)

**per serving:**
157 calories, 8 g protein, 29 g carbohydrates, 2 g fat, 0 mg cholesterol, 5 g dietary fiber, 58 mg sodium. High in dietary fiber, vitamin A (beta carotene), vitamin E, thiamine, riboflavin, niacin, vitamin $B_6$, vitamin $B_{12}$, vitamin C, folate, and pantothenic acid. A good source of protein, carbohydrate, vitamin D, calcium, magnesium, and potassium.

# nutritional yeast

Nutritional yeast, also known as brewer's yeast, is a nutritional supplement that's high in selenium and the B vitamins and can easily be added to your favorite food and beverage recipes. Unlike baker's yeast (the kind used in baking), nutritional yeast does not contain live yeast cultures. It is grown in purified molasses, under strict sanitary conditions and carefully regulated temperatures, then fermented, washed, pasteurized, and dried before it's sold in bags or jars at your local health food store. I like to use generic yeast flakes packaged in bags for my beverage recipes. It has a mild taste, and a competitive price.

## Health Claims For Cancer Prevention On Food Labels

Research confirming the link between diet and cancer convinced the Food and Drug Administration (FDA) to allow certain foods to carry labels with cancer-fighting claims. According to the 1990 Nutrition Labeling and Education Act, a food product may carry cancer-related health claims on its label if it is

- low in fat, containing 3 or fewer grams of fat per serving or 1 gram or less of saturated fat per serving and less than 95 mg of cholesterol per serving, or
- high in fiber, specifically containing a grain, fruit or vegetable that has 5 grams or more of fiber per serving.

Fruits and vegetables that are low in fat, high in fiber, and good sources of vitamins A or C can also be advertised as having cancer-fighting properties.

# Mango Milk
# with Green Tea

Combine mangoes, which are loaded with vitamins, and green tea, with its powerful antioxidants, and you've got a drink that can help fight cancer and heart disease. Try it as a midafternoon snack or as part of a healthy breakfast.

½ mango, cubed
½ cup one-percent milk or soy milk
1 cup green tea
dash nutmeg (garnish)

Combine the ingredients in a blender and process until smooth. Garnish with a dash of nutmeg.

**yield:**
  1 serving (2 cups)

**per serving with 1 percent milk:**
  118 calories, 5 g protein, 23 g carbohydrate, 2 g fat, 5 mg cholesterol, 2 g dietary fiber, and 64 mg sodium. High in vitamin A and carotenoids, riboflavin, vitamin $B_{12}$, vitamin C, vitamin D, and calcium. A good source of thiamine, vitamin $B_6$, vitamin E, and folate.

# Soy Peach Strawberry Smoothie

**Too tired to** fix a full meal? Try this energizing, nutrient-dense smoothie. Low in sodium, high in vitamin A and the B vitamins, and a good source of protein, dietary fiber, and magnesium, this drink is recommended for those with chronic fatigue syndrome. The soy protein base makes it an excellent choice for heart disease prevention, too.

$\frac{1}{2}$ cup fortified soy milk or skim or low-fat milk
1 peach, peeled and quartered, or $\frac{1}{2}$ cup frozen sliced
    peaches
3 strawberries, fresh or frozen
1 tablespoon wheat germ

Combine ingredients in blender and purée. Serve.

**yield:**
1 serving (1 cup)

**per serving:**
145 calories, 8 g protein, 23 g carbohydrates, 3 g fat, 0 cholesterol, 4 g dietary fiber, 53 mg sodium. High in vitamin A, thiamine, vitamin $B_{12}$, vitamin C, folate, and magnesium. A good source of protein, dietary fiber, riboflavin, niacin, vitamin $B_6$, vitamin D, pantothenic acid, calcium, iron, potassium, selenium and zinc.

# Creamy Orange Pineapple Refresher

Delicious any time, this tropical drink is particularly beneficial when you're suffering from a cold or bacterial infection. It packs a healthy dose of vitamin C, and live cultures in yogurt help replace beneficial bacteria that antibiotics can destroy. Wheat germ adds zinc, another cold fighter. (If you like the orange/pineapple flavor combination but are avoiding dairy, try the Orange Pineapple Refresher recipe on page 107.)

½ cup orange juice
½ cup fresh pineapple chunks or ½ cup of canned pineapple chunks (packed in unsweetened juice)
½ cup vanilla nonfat yogurt with live cultures
1 teaspoon wheat germ

Combine ingredients in a blender and process until smooth. Serve.

**yield:**
1 serving (1¼ cups)

**per serving:**
214 calories, 8 g protein, 45 g carbohydrates, 1 g fat, 2 mg cholesterol, 2 g dietary fiber, 86 mg sodium. High in riboflavin, vitamin C, calcium, and a good source of zinc, potassium, protein, carbohydrate, thiamine, vitamin $B_6$, vitamin $B_{12}$, folate, pantothenic acid, and magnesium.

# Prune-Raisin Smoothie

**Prunes and raisins** are soaked in hot water, then blended with yogurt and applesauce to create a fruity beverage that's high in antioxidants and an excellent aid for constipation. Fiber, of course, keeps things moving along the digestive tract, while the dihydroxphenylisatin in prunes is a bowel stimulant, and raisins contain tartaric acid, a natural laxative.

> 5 dried prunes, pitted
> $\frac{1}{4}$ cup raisins
> $\frac{3}{4}$ cup boiling or hot water
> $\frac{1}{4}$ cup plain nonfat yogurt
> $\frac{1}{4}$ cup unsweetened applesauce
> dash cinnamon

Soak prunes and raisins in boiling water. After 20 minutes, place in a blender and purée. Add the yogurt, applesauce, and cinnamon and purée again. Serve.

**yield:**
1 serving ($1\frac{1}{2}$ cups)

**per serving:**
286 calories, 6 g protein, 71 g carbohydrates, 1 g fat, 1 mg cholesterol, 5 g dietary fiber, 62 mg sodium. High in vitamin A, riboflavin, calcium, and potassium. A good source of protein, thiamine, niacin, vitamin $B_6$, vitamin $B_{12}$, vitamin E, copper, iron, and magnesium.

# Blueberry Smoothie

Here's to your heart health: magnesium, calcium, and potassium help keep blood pressure low; flaxseed contributes healthy omega-3 acids to lower unhealthy LDL cholesterol. And with a low-fat dairy base, this smoothie qualifies for the DASH (Dietary Approaches to Stop Hypertension) diet. What's more, the soy protein in the soy milk offers heart protection.

> 8 oz. container low-fat or nonfat blueberry yogurt (or one
> 8-ounce container vanilla yogurt plus $\frac{1}{3}$ cup fresh
> or unsweetened frozen blueberries)
> $\frac{1}{2}$ cup fortified soy milk
> 2 teaspoons ground flaxseed

Combine all ingredients in a blender and process until smooth, or mix well with a spoon or wire whip. Serve.

**yield:**
  1 serving ($1\frac{1}{3}$ cups)

**per serving (with blueberry yogurt):**
  316 calories, 16 g protein, 52 g carbohydrates, 3 g dietary fiber, 7 g fat, 2 g saturated fat, 10 mg cholesterol, 173 mg sodium. High in riboflavin, vitamin $B_{12}$, calcium. A good source of vitamin A, thiamine, vitamin E, folate, pantothenic acid, magnesium, potassium, selenium and zinc.

# Flaxseed

Flaxseed (which comes from flax, the plant used to make linen) can be ground in a coffee grinder and stirred into drinks for added nutritional benefits. Flaxseed is high in fiber and provides healthy omega-3 fatty acids, which can lower levels of "bad" LDL cholesterol. Also, flax and flaxseed contain lignans, powerful antioxidants that eliminate free radicals and help prevent heart disease, cancer, and menopause symptoms.

Flaxseed is best stored refrigerated or frozen.

# Soy Cantaloupe Smoothie

Similar in taste and color to the popular bottled soy drinks sold in melon, orange, and lime flavors, this smoothie makes a great introduction to soy. In addition to being delicious, it's high in the healing antioxidants (beta carotene, vitamin C, and vitamin E).

> ½ cup vanilla-flavored fortified soy milk
> ¼ cup orange juice
> ½ cup cubed cantaloupe, honeydew, or watermelon

Combine the ingredients in the blender and process until smooth.

**yield:**
   1 serving (1 cup)

**per serving:**
   131 calories, 4 g protein, 25 g carbohydrates, 2 g fat, 0 mg cholesterol, 1 g dietary fiber, 53 mg sodium. High in vitamin A, vitamin C, vitamin $B_{12}$, vitamin E, and folate. A good source of thiamine, vitamin $B_6$, vitamin D, calcium, magnesium, and potassium.

# Antioxidants

Antioxidants—vitamins C, E, and A, the mineral selenium, beta carotene and other carotenoids—are compounds found in fruits, vegetables, and whole grains that can actually help fight disease and aging. How do they do it? Antioxidants protect our bodies from free radicals—the oxygen molecules that are created naturally when our cells produce energy or (less naturally) when our bodies are exposed to harmful toxins in the environment. Left alone, free radicals can damage our healthy cells. Antioxidants bind with free radicals, preventing them from doing further damage.

Antioxidants are measured in units called an ORAC (Oxygen Radical Absorbance Capacity). Research has suggested that in order to reap the benefits of antioxidants, between 3,000 and 5,000 ORAC units should be consumed daily.

## fruits high in ORAC units (listed from highest to lowest ORAC content) per 100 g (3½ oz.)

| | |
|---|---|
| Prunes | 5770 |
| Raisins | 2830 |
| Blueberries | 2400 |
| Blackberries | 2036 |
| Strawberries | 1540 |
| Raspberries | 1220 |
| Plums | 949 |
| Oranges | 750 |
| Red grapes | 739 |
| Cherries | 670 |
| Kiwi | 602 |
| Pink grapefruit | 483 |

## vegetables high in ORAC units (listed from highest to lowest ORAC content) per 100 g (3½ oz.)

| | |
|---|---|
| Kale | 1770 |
| Spinach | 1260 |
| Brussels sprouts | 980 |
| Alfalfa sprouts | 930 |
| Broccoli | 890 |
| Beets | 840 |
| Red bell peppers | 710 |
| Onion | 450 |
| Corn | 400 |
| Eggplant | 390 |

# Psyllium Soother

**Try this fruity,** high-fiber drink for constipation relief. Active cultures found in lactose-free milk, acidophilus milk, and yogurt can also help relieve the symptoms of irritable bowel syndrome.

> 1 cup cubed cantaloupe
> ½ cup sliced strawberries
> ½ cup plain nonfat yogurt, lactose-free milk, or
>    acidophilus milk
> 1 teaspoon powdered psyllium

Combine ingredients in blender and purée. Serve immediately.

**yield:**
   1 serving (about 1½ cups)

**per serving with plain nonfat yogurt:**
   158 calories, 9 g protein, 32 g carbohydrates, 1 g fat, 2 mg cholesterol, 6 g dietary fiber, 110 mg sodium. High in vitamin A, dietary fiber, riboflavin, vitamin C, folate, calcium, and potassium. A good source of protein, carbohydrates, vitamin $B_6$, vitamin $B_{12}$, folate, magnesium, and zinc.

# psyllium

Psyllium, or psyllium seed, is a soluble fiber that may be helpful in lowering blood cholesterol and is recommended for hemorrhoids, irritable bowel syndrome, and constipation. Once ingested, psyllium absorbs water and helps soften stools as they pass through the digestive tract.

Psyllium is the active ingredient in "natural" over-the-counter laxatives such as Metamucil and can be found in some ready-to-eat cereals. You can also buy it in powdered form at health food stores and add it to your favorite beverage.

Some people are allergic to psyllium, so start with a teaspoon and work up to two teaspoons a day if needed. Mix each teaspoon of psyllium with at least $3/4$ cups of any liquid, and drink the mixture quickly before it has a chance to thicken. To ensure proper digestion, drink plenty of fluids when you add psyllium to your diet.

# Golden Quencher

Apricots are packed with nutrients, and so is this delicious drink. Beta carotene, which gives apricots their golden-orange color, helps protect against cancer, heart disease, and stroke. Apricots also contain malic acid, recommended to ease the symptoms associated with fibromyalgia. If you don't have ripe fresh apricots on hand, canned apricots or apricot nectar are an equally healthy alternative.

3 apricots, pitted and quartered or ½ cup apricot nectar
½ cup apple juice
½ cup fortified soy milk

Combine the ingredients in a blender. Purée. Serve.

**yield:**
1 serving (1½ cups)

**per serving:**
174 calories, 7 g protein, 33 g carbohydrates, 3 g dietary fiber, 3 g fat, 0 mg cholesterol, 57 mg sodium. High in vitamin A, vitamin B$_{12}$, and vitamin C. A good source of vitamin E, calcium, iron, magnesium, and potassium.

# Avocado Smoothie

This thick, pale green smoothie is nutrient-dense. Avocado and soy protein benefit the heart and blood pressure; orange juice adds vitamin C for healing. And because it's high in magnesium, this drink is recommended for persons with fibromyalgia and chronic fatigue syndrome.

$\frac{1}{2}$ ripe avocado
$\frac{1}{2}$ cup freshly squeezed orange juice
$\frac{1}{2}$ cup fortified soy milk

Remove the skin and the pit from the avocado; place the fruit in a blender. Add the orange juice and soy milk and process until smooth. Pour into a glass and serve.

**yield:**
1 serving ($1\frac{1}{2}$ cups)

**per serving:**
283 calories, 8 g protein, 27 g carbohydrate, 18 g fat, 10 g mono fat, 0 cholesterol, 5 g dietary fiber, 64 mg sodium. High in dietary fiber, vitamin A, thiamine, vitamin $B_6$, vitamin $B_{12}$, vitamin C, vitamin E, folate, magnesium and potassium. A good source of riboflavin, niacin, pantothenic acid, calcium, copper, and iron.

# avocado

Don't be scared off by the relatively high fat content in avocado-based drinks. Avocado is a healthy source of "good" monounsaturated fat, which can actually lower blood cholesterol. And half an avocado has more blood-pressure regulating potassium than a medium-size banana. If fat is an issue for you, look for Florida avocados, which contain about half the fat found in their California cousins. (Talk to your produce manager or look for stickers indicating state of origin.)

A ripe avocado is slightly soft—it should yield somewhat under gentle finger pressure. (Harder avocados will ripen in a few days at room temperature.) Store a ripe avocado in the refrigerator and use it as soon as possible. Once cut, an avocado will turn brown unless it is treated with lemon juice or tightly wrapped and refrigerated.

# Ginger Mango Supersmoothie

This is one powerful drink! Superhealer antioxidants (vitamins A, C, and E, beta carotene, and selenium) and live yogurt cultures give your immune system a terrific boost. Ginger adds kick and can help relieve migraine headaches, stomach distress, and motion sickness. And calcium, magnesium, and potassium help keep blood pressure low.

> 1 mango
> ½ cup plain nonfat yogurt
> ½ cup hot ginger tea, cooled (see page 177)
> ⅛ teaspoon ground nutmeg

Peel and core the mango and drop into a blender. Add the yogurt and ginger tea. Blend. Pour into a glass, adding ice if desired. Top with ground nutmeg.

**yield:**
1 serving (1 generous cup)

**per serving:**
205 calories, 8 g protein, 45 g carbohydrate, 1 g fat, 2 mg cholesterol, 4 g dietary fiber, 101 mg sodium. High in vitamin A, riboflavin, vitamin C, and calcium. A good source of protein, carbohydrate, fiber, thiamine, vitamin $B_6$, vitamin $B_{12}$, vitamin E, folate, pantothenic acid, copper, magnesium, potassium and selenium.

# Island Powerhouse

Tropical fruits are nutritional powerhouses—they're loaded with fiber, phytochemicals, and vitamins. This pineapple and papaya smoothie brings you a taste of the islands and a healthy dose of vitamin C. (To make your own fresh papaya purée, add peeled cubed papaya to the blender with 2–3 tablespoons of water and purée.)

$\frac{1}{3}$ cup papaya purée, fresh or bottled
$\frac{1}{3}$ cup pineapple juice
$\frac{1}{3}$ cup nonfat vanilla yogurt

Combine the ingredients in a bowl and mix well with a wire whip. Serve.

**yield:**
1 serving (1 cup)

**per serving:**
149 calories, 5 g protein, 33 g carbohydrates, 0.3 g fat, 1 mg cholesterol, 2 g dietary fiber, 59 mg sodium. High in vitamin A and vitamin C. A good source of riboflavin, folate, calcium, protein, carbohydrate and potassium.

# Morning Superstart

If you can't take time out for a full breakfast, this satisfying, nutrient-dense drink is for you. It contains all the ingredients of a typical American breakfast: fruit, juice, cereal, coffee, and dairy. Drink it on the run if you have to—you'll be glad you got off to a healthy start!

> 8 oz. container low-fat or nonfat coffee yogurt (or 8 oz. plain low-fat or nonfat yogurt plus 1 teaspoon powdered instant coffee)
> $\frac{1}{4}$ cup apricot nectar
> 2 fresh apricots, pitted, or 2 canned pitted apricots
> 2 tablespoons toasted wheat germ
> 1 teaspoon cocoa powder
> $\frac{1}{8}$ teaspoon cinnamon

Combine ingredients in a blender and process until smooth. Serve.

**yield:**
1 serving (2 cups)

**per serving with low-fat yogurt:**
321 calories, 17 g protein, 54 g carbohydrates, 5 g fat, 2 g saturated fat, 11 mg cholesterol, 4 g dietary fiber, 153 mg sodium. High in protein, vitamin A, thiamine, riboflavin, vitamin $B_{12}$, folate, calcium, magnesium, potassium, selenium, and zinc. A good source of carbohydrates, dietary fiber, vitamin $B_6$, vitamin C, vitamin E, pantothenic acid, copper, and iron.

# Chocolate Kiwi Surprise

Chocolate and kiwi? Try it and see! This rich-tasting smoothie is a delicious source of vitamin C, dietary fiber, and potassium. Like soy milk, rice milk can be purchased in 8-ounce and 1-quart boxes that are stored at room temperature until opening. Or make your own rice milk (see Rice Cure, p. 156). Because it's high in fiber and wheat- and dairy-free, this drink is a good choice for persons with irritable bowel syndrome.

> 1 cup (8 oz.) chocolate-flavored rice milk (or 1 cup plain rice milk plus 2–3 teaspoons of chocolate syrup)
> 1 kiwi, peeled
> 1 banana, cut into chunks

Combine ingredients in a blender and process until smooth. Serve.

**yield:**
1 serving (about 2 cups)

**per serving:**
325 calories, 3 g protein, 75 g carbohydrates, 4 g fat, 0 mg cholesterol, 7 g dietary fiber, 120 mg sodium. High in vitamin C, dietary fiber, carbohydrate, and potassium. A good source of vitamin E, folate, copper, and magnesium.

# Kiwi Soy Smoothie

**So simple, yet** so good for you! This smoothie is loaded with nutrients. It's a fine source of dietary fiber, too.

> 1 kiwi
>
> 1 cup fortified soy milk

Peel the kiwi, cut it into quarters and combine with the soy milk in a blender. Blend and serve.

**yield:**

1 serving (1 cup)

**per serving:**

176 calories, 11 g protein, 24 g carbohydrate, 4 g fat, 0 mg cholesterol, 3 g dietary fiber, 109 mg sodium. High in protein, vitamin A, vitamin C, vitamin $B_{12}$, vitamin E, calcium, magnesium, and potassium. A good source of dietary fiber, thiamine, vitamin $B_6$, vitamin D, folate, and iron.

# Kiwi Strawberry Smoothie

Add strawberries to the Kiwi Soy Smoothie and you'll get more than just delightful flavor. Strawberries add pantothenic acid, copper, and phytochemicals that strengthen the immune system. Try this one for relief of PMS symptoms—it's high in vitamin E, calcium, and magnesium. The vitamin $B_6$ and carbohydrates can also help relieve stress and regulate mood swings. With fructose for quick energy, it can even aid in hangover recovery.

> 1 ripe kiwi, peeled
> 1 cup fresh sliced strawberries
> 1 cup fortified soy milk
> 1 packet or ¾ teaspoon fructose

Add ingredients to blender, purée, and serve.

**yield:**
> 1 serving (2 cups)

**per serving :**
> 231 calories, 12 g protein, 37 g carbohydrates, 5 g fat, 0 cholesterol, 6 g dietary fiber, 111 mg sodium. High in dietary fiber, vitamin A, vitamin $B_{12}$, vitamin C, vitamin E, folate, calcium, magnesium, and potassium. A good source of carbohydrates, thiamine, riboflavin, vitamin $B_6$, vitamin D, pantothenic acid, copper, and iron.

# Mighty Blue Healer

The healing powers of this tasty blue drink are mighty indeed. It's brimming with healing phytochemicals and healthy B vitamins.

> ½ cup soy milk
> ½ cup fresh blueberries
> ¼ cup orange juice
> 1 teaspoon ground flaxseed, psyllium, or bran

Purée in blender and serve cold.

**yield:**

1 serving (1 cup)

**per serving:**

146 calories, 7 g protein, 25 g carbohydrates, 4 g fat, 0 cholesterol, 4 g dietary fiber, 58 mg sodium. High in vitamin $B_{12}$ and vitamin C. A good source of protein, dietary fiber, vitamin A, thiamine, vitamin E, folate, calcium, magnesium, and potassium.

# High-PO

High potassium, that is. One serving of this fruity pink drink supplies 900 mg of potassium, almost half the day's 2000 milligram requirement. Potassium helps prevent high blood pressure, promotes muscle contraction, and is important in maintaining the fluid and electrolyte balance in our cells. Try it for a midday pick-me-up.

1 ripe banana
6 strawberries
1 cup apple juice
4 teaspoons lemon or lime juice

Add ingredients to blender and blend. Serve.

**yield:**
1 serving ($1\frac{1}{2}$ cups)

**per serving:**
252 calories, 2 g protein, 64 g carbohydrates, 2 g fat, 0 cholesterol, 5 g dietary fiber, 10 mg sodium. High in carbohydrate, dietary fiber, vitamin $B_6$, and vitamin C, folate, and potassium. A good source of thiamine, riboflavin, iron, and magnesium.

# Pear-Blueberry Smoothie

This fruity, refreshing smoothie tastes so good you'll forget you are drinking something nutritious! And nutritious it is, with the healing power of blueberries, soy, and yogurt with live cultures. Sunflower seeds are a wonderful source of the antioxidant selenium and heart-healthy magnesium.

$\frac{1}{2}$ pear, peeled
$\frac{1}{2}$ cup blueberries
$\frac{1}{2}$ cup fortified soy milk
$\frac{1}{2}$ cup plain skim yogurt
1 tablespoon unsalted sunflower seeds

Combine the ingredients in a blender and purée. Serve.

**yield:**
1 serving ($1\frac{1}{2}$ cups)

**per serving:**
270 calories, 14 g protein, 41 g carbohydrates, 7 g fat, 2 mg cholesterol, 5 g dietary fiber, 151 mg sodium. High in protein, riboflavin, vitamin $B_{12}$, vitamin C, vitamin E, calcium, and potassium. A good source of dietary fiber, carbohydrate, vitamin A, thiamine, vitamin $B_6$, folate, pantothenic acid, copper, magnesium, selenium, and zinc.

# Soy Do It

Try this refreshing, light-green drink along with a few slices of whole-wheat toast for a healthy, well-rounded breakfast. With 40 milligrams of isoflavones, Soy Do It can help relieve menopausal symptoms and protect against heart disease. Calcium, potassium, and magnesium are good for your blood pressure, and tropical fruits provide fiber and immune-boosting vitamin C.

> 1 kiwi, peeled
> 1 cup fortified soy milk
> ½ cup fresh cubed pineapple
> ½ cup orange juice
> pineapple slice (for garnish)

Add ingredients to blender and purée. Garnish with pineapple slice.

**yield:**
1 serving (1½ cups)

**per serving:**
270 calories, 12 g protein, 47 g carbohydrate, 5 g fat, 0 cholesterol, 4 g dietary fiber, 111 mg sodium. High in protein, vitamin A, vitamin C, vitamin E, folate, calcium, magnesium, and potassium. A good source of carbohydrates, dietary fiber, vitamin D, copper, iron, and isoflavones.

# Purple Protein Power Shake

A high-protein drink can help you keep your mind on your work—try one or two servings of this purple shake for lunch, and see how you feel that afternoon. It may help elevate your mood, too: Vitamin $B_{12}$ and folate help your body convert the methionine found in soy into mood-enhancing SAMe.

> 1 cup vanilla fortified soy milk
> 1 cup (6 ounces) firm tofu
> 1 cup fresh or frozen, unthawed blueberries
> $\frac{1}{4}$ cup orange juice
> 2 scoops (6 tablespoons) soy protein powder (optional)

Combine all ingredients in a blender and process until smooth. Serve.

**yield:**
   2 servings ($1\frac{1}{2}$ cups each)

**per serving without protein powder:**
   221 calories, 13 g protein, 31 g carbohydrates, 5 g fat, 0 cholesterol, 2 g dietary fiber, 95 mg sodium. High in protein, vitamin $B_{12}$, vitamin C, and a good source of vitamin A, thiamine, folate, calcium, copper, iron, magnesium, and potassium.

**per serving with protein powder:**
   268 calories, 21 g protein, 36 g carbohydrate, 5 g fat, 0 cholesterol, 3 g dietary fiber, 96 mg sodium. High in protein, thiamine, vitamin $B_{12}$, vitamin C, folate, calcium, copper, iron, magnesium, phosphorus, potassium, and a good source of dietary fiber, vitamin A and zinc.

# Cocoa Fruit Smoothie

**This nutrient-dense** drink will fill you up and lift your spirits! Cocoa produces mood-enhancing endorphins, and vitamins $B_6$, $B_{12}$, and folate help your body produce SAMe from the methionine found in soy. With soy protein and lots of carbohydrates, this drink may help relieve PMS symptoms, as well.

> ½ banana, cut into chunks
> 1 peach, peeled and sliced, or 1 cup sliced peaches
>    (unsweetened frozen peaches or canned and
>    packed in juice)
> 2 teaspoons Dutch process cocoa powder
> 1 cup vanilla-flavored fortified soy milk

Combine all ingredients in a blender and purée until smooth.

**yield:**
   1 serving (1½ cups)

**per serving:**
   260 calories, 8 g protein, 50 g carbohydrates, 4 g fat, 0 mg cholesterol, 4 g dietary fiber, 92 mg sodium. High in vitamin A, dietary fiber, vitamin $B_6$, vitamin $B_{12}$, vitamin C, vitamin D, vitamin E, folate, calcium, magnesium, and potassium. A good source of protein, carbohydrates, thiamine, riboflavin, niacin, pantothenic acid, copper, and iron.

# Mellow Mama

Turn to dairy-free, soy-free Mellow Mama for relief from the stresses and symptoms of Premenstrual Syndrome. Fruits, vegetables, and nuts provide calming carbohydrates; the antioxidant vitamins A, C, and E are also recommended for PMS. Make your own almond milk (see page 151) or buy it at your local health food store.

$\frac{1}{2}$ cup raw spinach, washed and drained

1 orange, peeled and sectioned

$\frac{1}{4}$ cup almond milk

1 teaspoon honey

$\frac{1}{2}$ teaspoon lemon juice

$\frac{1}{4}$ teaspoon mustard

Combine all ingredients in a blender and purée until smooth.

**yield:**

1 serving

**per serving:**

123 calories, 3 g protein, 23 g carbohydrates, 3 g fat, 0 cholesterol, 4 g dietary fiber, 29 mg sodium. High in vitamin A, vitamin C, and a good source of fiber, vitamin E, folate, magnesium, and potassium.

**3**

Tea, whether green, black, or herbal, contains disease-fighting compounds and can often provide relief for specific ailments. Use loose tea leaves or convenient tea bags; blend different kinds of teas or add spices and juices to create new flavors. Soothing and hot or refreshing and iced, the teas in this chapter are healthy and easy to prepare.

# teas, tisanes, infusions, and coffees

# Lemon Balm
# Anxiety Reducer

A hot cup of tea, slowly prepared, held, and consumed, can do wonders to soothe the mind, body, and spirit. Lemon balm is particularly calming and can help with anxiety and insomnia.

> 2 teaspoons or 1 bag lemon balm tea
> 2 teaspoons or 1 bag chamomile tea
> 1 teaspoon or 1 bag peppermint tea
> 2 cups boiling water
> Ginger syrup (see page 176) or mint syrup (see page 178) to taste

Combine the teas in a cup or teapot. Pour boiling water over the tea and steep for 4 to 5 minutes. Strain. Add ginger or mint syrup to taste. Serve.

**yield:**
2 servings (1 cup each)

**per serving:**
2 calories, 0 protein, 1 g carbohydrate, 0 fat, 0 cholesterol, 0 dietary fiber, 2 mg sodium.

# infusions

An infusion is a term for a tea prepared by pouring boiling water over fresh or dried herbs. The hot water is infused with the essence of the herbs by steeping. An infusion and a tisane are the same.

# Doubly Green Tea

Cool and refreshing, this lime-green iced tea delivers a hefty dose of antioxidant polyphenols and 23 percent of the recommended Daily Value of vitamin C. This tea is also good for the heart and circulatory system; vitamin C may help lower cholesterol, while the bioflavonoids in lime and other citrus juices may protect the blood vessels and act as blood thinners.

> 1 cup boiling water
> 1–2 teaspoons loose green tea or 1 bag green tea
> 3 tablespoons lime juice
> 4 packets (3 teaspoons) fructose or 3 teaspoons sugar
>      or sugar substitute to taste
> ice

Pour the boiled water over the loose tea or tea bag; steep for 2 to 3 minutes. Strain and allow to cool. Pour the lime juice into a tall glass. Add the fructose, sugar, or sugar substitute and stir to dissolve. Add the green tea and stir again. Add ice to fill the glass. Serve.

**yield:**
> 1 serving (1 cup)

**per serving:**
> 57 calories, 0.2 g protein, 16 g carbohydrate, 0.1 g fat, 0 cholesterol, 0.2 g dietary fiber, 9 mg sodium. High in vitamin C.

# green tea

Green tea is believed to prevent cancer and heart disease, lower cholesterol, and even prevent tooth decay. To brew a perfect cup of green tea, bring 1 cup of water to a boil, then allow it to cool slightly before pouring it over 1 to 2 teaspoons of tea leaves or a tea bag. (Loose green tea generally produces a stronger brew than a tea bag will.) Let the tea steep for just one or two minutes before straining it.

If you make green tea often, consider buying a small, Japanese-style teapot with a built-in strainer—it's a marvelous time-saver. In Japan, green tea leaves are reused for second cups or pots of tea; they're just steeped a bit longer the second time around.

# the power of polyphenols

Both green and black teas contain powerful polyphenols, antioxidants thought to prevent cancer and heart disease. But the polyphenols in green tea are more plentiful and easier for our bodies to absorb, earning green tea its star polyphenol status.

You can get your polyphenols by drinking hot, iced, or caffeine-free green tea. Bottled green tea-based beverages contain fewer polyphenols, but they do deliver some.

# Echinacea Tea
# with Lemon and Honey

Next time you have a cold, try this soothing, immune-boosting tea. In fact, drink a cup at least three times a day until you're feeling better. Hot tea and honey will heat you up, make you sweat, and relieve throat pain and discomfort. Echinacea is particularly noted for its ability to fight infections and may lessen the intensity and duration of a cold. It also helps clear mucous from the throat. Echinacea does dry out your mouth and nasal passages, so drink more water and juices when taking echinacea.

To make a basic echinacea tea, pour one cup of boiling water over 2 teaspoons of dried echinacea and steep for 3 to 5 minutes. Add other herbs and spices for improved flavor.

> 2 cups boiling water
> 1 tablespoon loose echinacea or 1 bag echinacea tea
> 1 teaspoon peppermint tea or 1 bag peppermint tea
> 1 teaspoon dried chamomile flowers or 1 bag chamomile tea
> 1 teaspoon honey
> 2 teaspoons fresh lemon juice

Pour boiling water over the loose tea or tea bags and steep for 3 to 5 minutes. Remove bags or strain, then add the honey and lemon. Sip this tea while it's hot—the heat is helpful in healing as well.

**yield:**
2 servings (1 cup each)

**per serving:**
23 calories, 0 protein, 6 g carbohydrates, 0 fat, 0 cholesterol, 0 dietary fiber, 7 mg sodium.

# Licorice Root Soother

**Licorice root contains** glycyrrhizic acid, a decongestant that helps reduce inflammation and loosen mucous, making this an excellent tea for colds, cough, or bronchitis. Experts also believe that licorice root may be responsible for the production of interferon, which helps our bodies fight off infections.

Despite its name, licorice root is flavorless on its own; the fennel seed in this recipe produces that traditional "licorice" flavor. Fennel is a soothing spice, as are cardamom and cinnamon.

**Caution:** Licorice root can raise blood pressure and should not be taken by those on blood pressure medication. Excessive amounts of licorice root—more than 2 ounces a day—can be harmful for persons with liver disease or chronic hepatitis, those taking diuretics or steroids, and pregnant women.

> 1 bag licorice root tea or 1 dried licorice root stick
> 3–4 dried mint leaves or 1–2 teaspoons dried mint or 1 bag mint tea
> $\frac{1}{4}$ teaspoon crushed fennel seed
> pinch cardamom
> pinch cinnamon
> 1 cup water
> 1 teaspoon honey

If you're using a licorice root tea bag: Place the tea bag in a mug, along with the mint, fennel, cardamom, cinnamon. Add boiling water and let steep for 3 to 5 minutes. Strain. Add honey, mix well, and serve.

If you're using dried licorice root stick: Break one 4–inch dried licorice root stick into inch-long pieces. Place the pieces in 2 cups of water and bring to a boil; lower the heat and simmer for 15 minutes. Strain tea and pour one cup off into a cup or teapot. Add mint, fennel, cardamom, and cinnamon, then steep for 3 to 5 minutes. Add honey, mix well, and serve.

**yield:**
1 serving (1 cup)

**per serving:**
2 calories, 0 protein, 0.3 g carbohydrate, 0 fat, 0 cholesterol, 0 dietary fiber, 2 mg sodium.

# decoctions

Herbal decoctions are made by boiling herbs in water to extract their flavors and essences. The decoction method is used when making tea from dried twigs or roots.

# Greenberry Tea

Fruit-leaf teas are easy to prepare and can help alleviate digestive problems. To make a basic fruit-leaf tea, steep blackberry, blueberry, or raspberry leaves in boiling water for 5 minutes, strain, and serve. In this recipe, berry leaves are teamed with antioxidant-rich green tea to boost your immune system and soothe your stomach. (This tea can help stop diarrhea, too.)

> 1 cup boiling water
> 1 teaspoon green tea leaves or 1 bag green tea
> 1–2 teaspoons dried blackberry, blueberry, or raspberry
>     leaves
> 1–2 teaspoons fruit syrup (optional)

Pour boiling water over the leaves or tea bag and steep for 3 to 5 minutes. Strain. Serve. One or two teaspoons of fruit syrup can be added for sweetening and flavor if desired.

**yield:**
   1 serving (1 cup)

**per serving:**
   2 calories, 0 protein, 0.5 g carbohydrates, 0 fat, 0 cholesterol, 0 dietary fiber, 2 mg sodium.

# echinacea

The herb echinacea (eh-kin-AY-shee-a), which comes from the purple coneflower, is believed to fight infection and boost the immune system. The species *echinacea purpurea* has also been shown to help fight urinary tract infections and to reestablish white blood cell count after cancer treatment.

Do not take or drink echinacea in any form if you are allergic to coneflowers, or if you have multiple sclerosis, AIDS, tuberculosis, leukemia or autoimmune diseases like rheumatoid arthritis and lupus.

# Watermelon Chamomile Frosty

This summer refresher delivers the healing powers of chamomile and the vitamin C of watermelon. And it tastes great, too! To make frozen watermelon cubes, freeze puréed watermelon in ice cube trays. The ice cubes can be stored in sealed plastic bags in the freezer. Keep a cold pitcher of chamomile tea in the refrigerator and making this drink is a snap.

**Caution:** Chamomile allergies can develop if you are allergic to ragweed.

    ½ cup chamomile tea, cooled
    1 cup frozen watermelon cubes
    1 teaspoon psyllium powder
    2 teaspoons mint syrup (optional, see page 178)

Start with cooled tea so it won't melt the frozen watermelon cubes. Pour cool tea into a blender with the frozen watermelon cubes. Puree and add psyllium, blend again, and serve immediately. Add mint syrup if desired.

This recipe can be doubled or tripled successfully.

**yield:**
    1 serving (1½ cups)

**per serving:**
    59 calories, 1 g protein, 15 g carbohydrates, 1 g fat, 0 mg cholesterol, 3 g dietary fiber, 6 mg sodium. High in vitamin C. A good source of dietary fiber, vitamin A, and vitamin B$_6$.

# chamomile

Calming chamomile can help bronchitis, colds, cough, fever, sore throat, and inflammation. It is also used to promote a good night's sleep. Hot chamomile tea also alleviates cramping and eases the associated discomfort of diarrhea.

To make basic chamomile tea, place 1 to 2 teaspoons of dried chamomile or one chamomile tea bag in a pot or mug. Add one cup of boiling water and steep for 3 to 5 minutes. Strain and serve.

# Basil Tea

Drink a cup of this basil tea before a meal to reduce gas or have one after a meal to aid digestion. Basil contains eugenol, a compound that may help reduce muscle spasms and ease cramps and other forms of stomach distress.

This is a strong tea, so don't let it steep too long. I like its clean flavor, but you might try adding peppermint or spearmint for a gentler taste. Or add stomach-friendly lactose-free milk to sweeten it. If gas is a problem, steer clear of sugar or honey.

> 1–2 teaspoons dried basil or 3–4 leaves fresh basil
> 1 cup boiling water
> lactose free milk (optional)

Pour boiling water over the basil and steep for 8–10 minutes. Strain and serve.

**yield:**
1 serving (1 cup)

**per serving:**
2 calories, 0 protein, 0 carbohydrate, 0 fat, 0 cholesterol, 0 dietary fiber, 0 sodium.

# tisanes

A tisane (ti-ZAN) is a French name for a tea made from an infusion of fresh or dried herbs. Alice Waters, owner of Chez Panisse restaurant and café in Berkeley, California, is renowned for the tisanes she serves. She pours very hot water over fresh herbs and allows them to steep for 4 or 5 minutes. Fresh herbal tisanes are beautiful prepared in a glass pot and served in glass teacups.

# Spirit-Lifting
# St. John's Wort Tea

Acting much like the commercial drug Prozac and related antidepressants, St. John's Wort is believed to enhance the serotonin level in the brain and relieve feelings of depression. Fortified soy milk in this recipe adds not only flavor but also carbohydrates, vitamin $B_6$, and vitamin $B_{12}$—all depression fighters—plus the antioxidant vitamin E.

Try a cup of this tea daily and see how you feel. If you don't detect improvement within a month, stop drinking it.

**Caution:** Do not take St. John's Wort if you are taking Nardil or other MAO inhibitors, the HIV medicine Indavir, of the transplant drug Cyclosporin, or birth control medication, as there can be a loss of therapeutic effect.

> 2 teaspoons St. John's Wort or 1 bag St. John's Wort tea
> 1 cup boiling water
> $1/4$ cup plain fortified soy milk
> $1/2$ teaspoon honey

Pour boiling water over the herb or tea bag and steep for 2 to 3 minutes. Strain or remove the bag; add the soy milk and honey. Serve.

**yield:**
1 serving ($1\frac{1}{4}$ cup)

**per serving:**
45 calories, 3 g protein, 7 g carbohydrate, 1 g fat, 0 cholesterol, 0 dietary fiber, 28 mg sodium. High in vitamin $B_{12}$. A good source of vitamin E.

# Iced Mochaccino

You'll probably agree that there are times when coffee and caffeine are appropriate. In the middle of the day, when energy ebbs, there is nothing like a cup of coffee. I love the smell of coffee in the morning, and reading the morning paper while holding and sipping from a warm mug is one of life's little pleasures.

Coffee can help relieve the tiredness and headache associated with a hangover. Iced Mochaccino contains several hangover helpers: caffeine (in the strong coffee and chocolate), fructose (in the chocolate syrup and whipped topping) and ice, which can provide headache relief by helping dilated blood vessels contract.

    1 cup strong coffee
    2 tablespoons chocolate syrup
    2 teaspoons powdered egg white (see page 34)
    2 tablespoons warm water
    2 packages fructose or 1½ teaspoons powdered
        fructose
    ice
    milk or cream as needed or preferred

Prepare strong coffee by using twice the amount of coffee grounds you usually use when brewing coffee—use 2 tablespoons of coffee for every cup of water. Combine one cup of brewed coffee and the chocolate syrup in a tall glass. Stir, and add ice to fill the glass.

In a bowl, combine warm water and the powdered egg white (do not use fresh, uncooked egg white, which can carry salmonella). Stir slowly for 2 minutes, allowing the egg white to absorb the water. Use a wire whip to beat until foamy; add the fructose and continue whipping until it is absorbed. Pour this froth into the glass of iced mochaccino and serve.

### yield:
1 serving (1 cup)

### per serving:
146 calories, 5 g protein, 31 g carbohydrates, 0.4 g fat, 0 cholesterol, 1 g dietary fiber, 81 mg sodium, 146 mg caffeine. A good source of protein and carbohydrates.

# fructose

Try using powdered or crystalline fructose to sweeten beverages when you want a quick burst of energy. Your body can absorb fructose, the sugar found naturally in fruit and in honey, more quickly than it can absorb sucrose, or table sugar. Fructose is one and a half times as sweet as table sugar, so you won't need to use as much.

# Green Ginger Tea

Add zing to a cup of healing green tea with spicy fresh ginger. Because it contains caffeine, this tea is also a good choice if you have a headache. Use a special ginger grater, sold in Asian markets, to grate your ginger. Or chop or slice the ginger then mince it in a garlic press.

> 1 teaspoon grated or minced fresh ginger or $\frac{1}{4}$ teaspoon powdered ginger
> 1–2 teaspoons loose green tea or 1 bag green tea
> 1 cup boiling water, cooled slightly
> sugar or honey to taste

Add the fresh or dried ginger and the green tea to a mug. Pour slightly cooled water over the tea and steep for 2 to 4 minutes. Strain if you're using the loose tea, and add sugar or honey to taste. Serve immediately or chill and serve over ice.

**yield:**
1 serving (1 cup)

**per serving:**
2 calories, 0 protein, 0.3 g carbohydrates, 0 fat, 0 cholesterol, 0 dietary fiber, 7 mg sodium.

# Aromatic Astragalus Tea

**Astragalus root,** a popular herb in Chinese medicine, is an immune system booster that's believed to increase the production of T-cells, which are among the body's first lines of defense against disease. Astragalus root is useful in combating colds and flu and in treating fatigue, arthritis and diarrhea. You can buy astragalus in convenient tea bag form, or prepare your own tea by placing one tablespoon of astragalus root (found in Chinese markets) in 1 cup of water and boiling for 15 to 20 minutes.

The herb has an unusual odor—it smells somewhat like cooked corn silk. In this recipe it is combined with jasmine tea, which adds a pleasant aromatic quality and antioxidant flavonoids. The echinacea in this tea helps fight colds or infection as well.

> 1 bag astragalus tea
> 1–2 teaspoons jasmine tea or 1 bag jasmine tea
> 1–2 teaspoons dried loose echinacea
> 1 cup boiling water

Pour the boiling water over the teas and steep for 2 to 3 minutes. Remove the bags and strain the tea. Serve with honey if desired.

**yield:**
1 serving (1 cup)

**per serving:**
2 calories, 0 protein, 0 carbohydrates, 0 fat, 0 cholesterol, 0 dietary fiber, 0 sodium.

# Green Tea with Punch

This healthful punch combines two heavy-hitting immune system boosters, green tea and vitamin C (you'll get 40 milligrams in each serving). It promotes heart health, as well: green tea can help lower blood pressure and reduce the risk of stroke.

2 cups boiling water, slightly cooled
2 teaspoons loose green tea or 2 bags of green tea
2 cups cranberry juice
2¼ cups pineapple juice
ice

Prepare the tea by pouring the slightly cooled water over the tea or tea bags in a pot or bowl. Steep for 4 minutes, then strain and cool. Add the cranberry juice and pineapple juice to the cooled tea. Serve over ice.

**yield:**
    6 servings (about 1 cup each)

**per serving:**
    101 calories, 0.3 g protein, 25 g carbohydrates, 0 cholesterol, 0.3 g dietary fiber, 5 mg sodium. High in vitamin C.

# Passion Flower
# Bedtime Tea

**Try a cup of** this calming, aromatic tea about thirty minutes before bedtime. Passion flower, which grows naturally on vines in the southeastern United States and south to Brazil and Argentina, is known for its soothing properties. This tea will reduce anxiety and ensure a good night's sleep.

> 1 cup boiling water
> 1 bag passion flower tea
> 1 teaspoon dried lemon balm
> 1 teaspoon honey

Pour the boiling water over the tea and steep for 3 to 5 minutes (for a stronger taste, steep up to 10 minutes). Strain or remove the tea bag, add honey, and serve.

**yield:**
   1 serving (1 cup)

**per serving:**
   23 calories, 0 protein, 6 g carbohydrates, 0 fat, 0 cholesterol, 0 dietary fiber, 3 mg sodium.

# Grandmom Rose's Cup of Tea

My grandmother had two favorite cures for insomnia: the bottle of blackberry brandy she kept in her closet and this drink, which she called her "cup of tea." She drank this every night, after she set the table for breakfast. I always wondered why she called it tea—there isn't a drop of tea in it. Regardless, it seemed to do the trick!

    1 cup boiling water
    2–3 tablespoons low-fat or skim milk

Combine in a mug and sip slowly.

**yield:**
    1 serving (1 cup)

**per serving with low-fat milk:**
    13 calories, 1 g protein, 2 g carbohydrates, 0.3 g fat, 1 mg cholesterol, 0 dietary fiber, 23 mg sodium.

# Soothing
# Spearmint Tea

A patch of spearmint grows in my summer garden, and I'm always surprised at the number of people who recognize it and pull off a leaf to chew. Enjoy this chamomile and spearmint tea after dinner. Spearmint leaves have long been considered a folk remedy for gas. The fennel seeds help humor the stomach and are particularly recommended for those with irritable bowel syndrome.

**Caution:** People with allergies to ragweed and its relatives should avoid chamomile.

> ½ teaspoon fennel seeds, toasted or untoasted
> 2 teaspoons chamomile or 1 bag chamomile tea
> 2–3 teaspoons of spearmint tea leaves or 1 bag
>       spearmint tea
> 1 cup boiling water
> 1 teaspoon mint syrup, if desired

Crush the fennel seeds and combine with chamomile and spearmint tea leaves or bags in a cup. Add boiling water and steep for 3 to 4 minutes. Strain and serve.

**yield:**
   1 serving (1 cup)

**per serving (estimated):**
   15 calories, 1 g protein, 2 g carbohydrates, 0 fat, 0 cholesterol, 0 dietary fiber, 12 mg sodium.

# fennel seeds

Fennel seeds, which have an anise or licorice-like flavor, are believed to hasten digestion and are among the seeds traditionally chewed after meals in India. Buy fennel seeds in the spices section of your supermarket. For better flavor, try toasting them: Place seeds in a dry skillet and heat for a minute or two, stirring to prevent burning. Cool the seeds and store them in a sealed container.

To make a basic fennel tea, pour one cup of boiling water (or hot milk) over toasted fennel seeds. Steep for 10 minutes. Strain the tea and drink it before meals.

# moroccan spearmint tea

Esther Press McManus, now a chef and cooking teacher in Philadelphia, tells me that sugar-sweetened spearmint tea is a popular cure-all in her native Morocco. In her favorite recipe, McManus combines spearmint tea with green tea and adds dried verbena from her garden.

# Grape Tea

You could be traditional and add water to your frozen grape juice concentrate. But for added phytochemicals *and* great taste, why not use green tea instead? Tangy Grape Tea is refreshing and packed with immune-system strengtheners.

> 36 oz brewed green tea (three 12-ounce frozen-juice cans full of tea)
> 12 oz. frozen grape juice

Prepare the juice by mixing grape concentrate with three cans (36 ounces) of green tea. Mix well and serve cold.

**yield:**
   12 servings (½ cup each)

**per serving:**
   52 calories, 0.2 g protein, 13 g carbohydrates, 0 fat, 0 cholesterol, 0 dietary fiber, 5 mg sodium. High in vitamin C.

# Heart Soothing Chai

Spicy chai (pronounced *ch-eye*), a beverage hailing from the Himalayan mountain regions of Asia, is a rich-tasting mixture of tea, spices, milk, and sugar. Commercial chai can be heavily sweetened and is usually made with black tea. Instead, try this heart-healthy version, made with green tea and soy milk. Serve it hot, or cold over ice.

½ cup water
3 crushed allspice seeds
3 cloves, crushed
pinch cinnamon
pinch powdered ginger
1 bag or 1–2 teaspoons loose green tea
½ cup fortified vanilla-flavored soy milk
½–1 teaspoon brown sugar or honey

Pour the water in a cup and add the allspice, cloves, cinnamon, and ginger. Microwave for 1 minute on high power. Remove from the microwave and add the tea bag or green tea; steep for 2 to 3 minutes, then strain. Add the soy milk and brown sugar. Serve.

To make this tea without a microwave, mix the spices with the water and bring to a boil on the stove. Place 1 to 2 teaspoons of green tea or a tea bag in a small pot or cup; pour the spiced water over the tea and steep for several minutes. Strain, add the soy milk and brown sugar, and serve.

Chai can be served warm or over ice.

**yield:**
1 serving (1 cup)

**per serving with vanilla-flavored soy milk:**
85 calories, 3 g protein, 14 g carbohydrates, 2 g fat, 0 cholesterol, 0 dietary fiber, 50 mg sodium. High in vitamin $B_{12}$ and vitamin E. A good source of vitamin A, vitamin D, folate, and calcium.

# Lemongrass Ginger Tea

The inspiration for this mild, relaxing tea comes from the *True Thai* cookbook, written by Theresa Volpe Laursen, her husband Byron, and Victor Sodsook, a Thai chef and the owner of the Siamese Princess restaurant in Los Angeles. You can find fresh lemongrass at Asian groceries, but use the dried variety if you must. Crystallized ginger imparts a nice flavor. This tea is also delicious iced.

> 1 inch of fresh lemongrass, thinly sliced, or 1 teaspoon dried lemongrass
> 1 piece of crystallized ginger, about 1 inch square
> 1 cup boiling water

Place the sliced lemongrass in a cup. Cut the ginger into smaller pieces and add to the cup. Pour the boiling water over both and steep for 5 minutes. (If you're using dried lemongrass, steep a bit longer, up to 15 minutes, to extract the most flavor). Strain and serve.

**yield:**
1 serving (1 cup)

**per serving (estimated):**
13 calories, 0 protein, 3 g carbohydrates, 0 fat, 0 cholesterol, 0 dietary fiber, 8 mg sodium.

# 4

The cold, sparkling cocktails in this chapter, made with seltzer or naturally sparking water, range from light, fruity beverages suitable for an evening soiree to sweet, soothing drinks that are perfect for those with an upset stomach. I've included some vegetable juice cocktails, brimming with vitamins and minerals, as well.

cocktails

and other sparkling beverages

# Tomato Cocktail

Made with fortified soy milk, this smooth cocktail contains 4 milligrams of iron—more than one-quarter of the recommended Daily Value for women. The vitamin C in the tomatoes helps our bodies absorb the nonheme (plant-derived) iron they also contain. The healthy fat in olive oil helps us absorb the antioxidant found in tomatoes, lycopene.

> 8 oz. stewed tomatoes, canned, no salt
> ¼ cup plain nonfat yogurt or fortified soy milk
> ½ teaspoon blackstrap molasses
> ¼ teaspoon olive oil

Combine all the ingredients in a blender and process until smooth. Serve over ice.

**yield:**
1 serving (1 cup)

**per serving (with yogurt):**
117 calories, 5 g protein, 20 g carbohydrates, 1 g fat, 1 mg cholesterol, 4 g dietary fiber, 76 mg sodium. High in vitamin C, calcium, iron, and a good source of dietary fiber, vitamin A, riboflavin, vitamin $B_{12}$, and potassium.

# Orange Ginger Quencher

Keep a jar of the base for this light, refreshing drink in the refrigerator so it's ready for adding the seltzer when you are on a hot summer day. It's high in healing vitamin C and contains spicy ginger to soothe the stomach. Ginger can be minced using a ginger grater (available in Asian markets) or a garlic press.

1 teaspoon minced ginger
1 cup boiling water
2 teaspoons sugar or honey (or less according to taste)
½ cup orange juice
1 cup seltzer

Place minced ginger in a cup. Pour the boiling water over the ginger and steep for 5 minutes. Strain and pour the ginger tea into a pitcher. Stir in the sugar, add ice, and stir once more. Then add the orange juice and seltzer. Stir and serve.

**yield:**
4 servings (½ cup each)

**per serving:**
22 calories, 0.2 g protein, 5 g carbohydrates, 0.1 g fat, 0 cholesterol, 0 dietary fiber, 13 mg sodium. High in vitamin C.

# UTI Cocktail

A mixture of baking soda and water is a popular folk remedy for bladder and urinary tract infections. Drink a UTI cocktail and call your doctor at the first signs of a urinary tract or bladder infection (pain and burning when urinating, frequent urination, passing blood, or voiding only small amounts). Don't drink this cocktail on a full stomach or if you're on a low-sodium diet. For additional relief, add baking soda to a bath and soak in it for a few minutes.

½ teaspoon baking soda
1 cup water

Combine the baking soda and water. Serve immediately.

**yield:**
1 serving (1 cup)

**per serving:**
0 calories, 0 protein, 0 carbohydrate, 0 dietary fiber, 0 cholesterol, 636 mg sodium.

# Cranberry Fizz

This sparkling drink is light and delicious. With antioxidant vitamin C and cancer-fighting ellagic acid, cranberry juice is a wonderful immune-system booster. Cranberry juice can help prevent urinary tract infections, too.

1 cup cranberry juice
¼ cup sparkling water or seltzer
1 teaspoon lemon juice
Ice
Lemon slice (garnish)

Combine cranberry juice, sparkling water or seltzer, and lemon juice in a glass. Stir and add ice and a lemon slice.

**yield:**
1 serving (1¼ cup)

**per serving:**
146 calories, 0 g protein, 37 g carbohydrate, 0.3 g fat, 0 cholesterol, 0.3 g dietary fiber, 7 mg sodium. High in vitamin C.

## and cranberry juice cocktail

Check product labels to see how much cranberry juice is in your cranberry juice cocktail. Cranberry juice has to be sweetened to make it palatable. Some cranberry juice cocktails contain only 27 percent juice, and many others contain even less. Look for a cocktail that lists cranberry juice as the first or second ingredient (often, high-fructose corn syrup will be listed first). If cranberry juice or cocktail is too acidic for your stomach, try diluting it with water.

# Frosty Apricot Mint Cooler

This drink provides 35 percent of the recommended Daily Value of vitamin A and 50 percent of the Daily Value of vitamin C. It's low in calories and thirst-quenching, too. Don't forget to eat the mint garnish—it contains anti-cancer compounds.

> ¾ cup (6 ounces/180 ml) apricot nectar
> ½ cup seltzer or sparkling water (no sodium)
> Mint garnish

Combine the apricot nectar and seltzer in a glass. Garnish with mint.

**yield:**
1 serving (1¼ cups)

**per serving:**
95 calories, 1 g protein, 25 g carbohydrates, 0.2 g fat, 0 cholesterol, 1 g dietary fiber, 6 mg sodium. High in vitamin A, carotenoids, and vitamin C (if fortified).

# apricots

Choose deep orange-gold apricots without green spots—the darker and brighter they are, the more beta-carotene and other carotenoids they contain. Ripe apricots are firm but give slightly when finger pressure is applied. Apricots can be ripened on the counter, but once ripe should be stored in the refrigerator.

Fresh apricot purée is delicious, high in dietary fiber, and can be diluted with seltzer or sparkling water to suit your taste. To make apricot purée, remove the pits from four to six apricots. Purée the apricots in a blender with 2 to 3 tablespoons of water. Or simply purée ¾ cup canned, juice-packed apricots along with 2 to 3 tablespoons of their juices.

# Blackberry Sparkle

Reach for a Blackberry Sparkle instead of a soda. It's low in calories and contains no artificial sweeteners, caffeine, or sodium. And unlike soda, it's low in phosphates, which can rob your body of calcium. Blackberries provide your body with ellagic acid, which may help prevent cancer.

> 2 tablespoons blackberry syrup (see page 182)
> ¾ cup seltzer or sparkling water
> Ice

Pour the syrup into a glass. Add the seltzer and stir. Serve over ice.

**yield:**
1 serving (¾ cup)

**per serving:**
105 calories, 0 g protein, 26 g carbohydrates, 0 g fat, 0 mg cholesterol, 0 g dietary fiber, 2 mg sodium. High in copper. A good source of vitamin C.

# Orange Pineapple Refresher

**While your friends** are sipping their cocktails, you can sip this nonalcoholic drink. Tropical fruit juices make it high in vitamin C. For a sophisticated touch, serve Orange-Pineapple Refresher in an interesting glass with a fresh pineapple triangle.

> ½ cup orange juice
> ½ cup pineapple chunks
> ¼ cup granulated sugar or 2 tablespoons sugar syrup
>     (see page 175)
> 2 tablespoons fresh lemon juice
> 1 cup sparkling water
> Pineapple slices (for garnish)

In a blender combine the orange juice, pineapple chunks, granulated sugar or sugar syrup, and lemon juice. Process until the pineapple is smooth. Divide between two glasses; add ½ cup sparkling water to each and stir. Serve garnished with pineapple slices.

**yield:**
    2 servings (1 cup each)

**per serving:**
    148 calories, 1 g protein, 38 g carbohydrates, 0.3 g fat, 0 mg cholesterol, 1 g dietary fiber, 3 mg sodium. High in vitamin C.

# Lemon Aid

Drink this one when you have a cold or the flu. It's based on an old folk remedy I learned from my friend Luis, who is originally from the Dominican Republic. If you like, add 2 teaspoons of raspberry syrup (see page 185) and try a Raspberry Lemon Aid. Limonene, a phytochemical in lemon and citrus fruits, may help our bodies fight cancer.

> 1 cup boiling water
> 3–4 tablespoons freshly squeezed lemon juice or 1
>     lemon, quartered
> 3 teaspoons honey

Combine boiling water and lemon juice in a cup (or combine cool water and 2 lemon quarters in a mug and microwave for 1.5 minutes; squeeze the juice from the remaining 2 lemon quarters into the mug.) Stir in honey. Serve hot.

**yield:**
   1 serving (1 cup)

**per serving:**
   76 calories, 0.2 g protein, 21 g carbohydrates, 0 g fat, 0 cholesterol, 0.2 g dietary fiber, 8 mg sodium. High in vitamin C.

**Note:** For Raspberry Lemon Aid add 2 teaspoons of unsweetened Raspberry Syrup (see staples section) to the Lemon Aid.

**per serving:**
   110 calories, 0.2 g protein, 30 g carbohydrates, 0 fat, 0 cholesterol, 0.2 g dietary fiber, 9 mg sodium. High in vitamin C.

# Sy's Lime Rickey

**My husband, Sy,** likes to cool down after a game of tennis with a refreshing Lime Rickey. It's an excellent thirst quencher. When made with fructose and served icy cold, it would also be good for a hangover.

> 3 tablespoons lime juice
> 4 packages or 1 tablespoon fructose, 1 tablespoon sugar or 3–4 packages non-caloric sweetener
> 1 cup sparkling water, spring water, or seltzer
> ice
> lime wedge or slice (for garnish)

Combine the lime juice and fructose or sweetener in a tall glass. Stir to dissolve. Add the sparkling water, spring water, or seltzer. Mix, then add enough ice to fill the glass. Garnish with a lime wedge or slice. Serve.

**yield:**
  1 serving (1 cup)

**per serving:**
  57 calories, 0.2 g protein, 16 g carbohydrates, 0 fat, 0 cholesterol, 0.2 g dietary fiber, 4 mg sodium. High in vitamin C.

# Quick Comeback

I developed the Quick Comeback for my friends who find tomato juice helpful when nursing a hangover. You don't have to have a hangover to enjoy it: it's low in calories, and high in lycopene and vitamins A and C. Canned vegetable juices can be high in sodium, so make sure you buy low-sodium V-8 for this drink. Nutritional yeast can be added for extra nutrition and flavor.

> 1 small can (5.5 oz.) low-sodium V-8
> ½ teaspoon unsulphured molasses
> 3 tablespoons plain nonfat yogurt
> ½ teaspoon nutritional yeast (optional)
> ice

Combine ingredients in a mug or glass. Stir, add ice, and serve.

**yield:**
1 serving (1 cup)

**per serving:**
74 calories, 4 g protein, 13 g carbohydrates, 0 g fat, 0.8 mg cholesterol, 2 g dietary fiber, 128 mg sodium. High in vitamin A and vitamin C. A good source of thiamine, riboflavin, vitamin $B_{12}$, folate, calcium, and iron.

# Strawberry Wine Cooler

According to the National Institutes of Health, moderate alcohol intake (no more than two glasses of wine a day) has been associated with a decreased risk of heart disease and stroke. In moderation (no more than two glasses a day), it can also help lower blood cholesterol. That's reason enough to try this sparkling strawberry cooler.

> 2 tablespoons fresh strawberry juice or 1 tablespoon
>     strawberry syrup
> ¼ cup red dry wine
> ½ cup sparkling water or seltzer
> ice

Strawberry juice is prepared by juicing whole fresh strawberries. About 4 large strawberries will yield 2 tablespoons of juice. Combine the juice, wine and sparkling water in a glass. Serve over ice.

**yield:**
    1 serving (¾ cup)

**per serving:**
    51 calories, 0.3 g protein, 3 g carbohydrates, 0 g fat, 0 g cholesterol, 0 g dietary fiber, 4 mg sodium. A good source of vitamin C.

# Blackberry Wine Cooler

This wine cooler looks and tastes like a festive holiday punch. Use a blackberry syrup made from real berries and sugar (see page 182) to get the healthful benefits of berries. Red wine and berries both contain ellagic acid, a cancer-fighting flavonoid.

> 1 tablespoon blackberry syrup
> 2 tablespoons water
> $\frac{1}{4}$ cup dry red wine
> $\frac{1}{4}$ cup sparkling water

Combine ingredients and serve over ice.

**yield:**
1 serving ($\frac{1}{2}$ cup)

**per serving:**
52 calories, 0 protein, 3 g carbohydrates, 0 g fat, 0 cholesterol, 0.3 g dietary fiber, 7 mg sodium.

# Tummy Rescue Remedy

Sweet, soothing, and perfect for relieving the symptoms of stomach flu. Ginger soothes the digestive system, while cranberry juice adds phytochemicals and vitamin C to strengthen the immune system.

> 2 tablespoons homemade ginger syrup (see p. 176)
> $\frac{2}{3}$ cup bottled cranberry juice cocktail

Combine the ginger syrup and cranberry juice cocktail in a glass. Serve over ice.

**yield:**
1 serving ($\frac{2}{3}$ cup)

**per serving:**
99 calories, 0 protein, 25 g carbohydrates, 0 fat, 0 cholesterol, 0 dietary fiber, 4 mg sodium. High in vitamin C.

# Homemade Ginger Ale

Making your own ginger ale is easy when you keep ginger syrup on hand. It contains fewer calories and more real ginger than you'll find in commercial ginger ales. I find it tastes better, too!

> $\frac{1}{4}$ cup ginger syrup (see page 176)
> $\frac{1}{2}$ cup seltzer or club soda
> ice
> 1 slice of lemon or lime (for garnish)

Pour the syrup into a glass and add the seltzer or club soda. Stir. Add ice and slice of lemon or lime. Serve.

**yield:**
  1 serving ($\frac{3}{4}$ cup)

**per serving:**
  34 calories, 0.3 g protein, 8 g carbohydrates, 0 g fat, 0 mg cholesterol, 0.3 g dietary fiber, 7 mg sodium.

# Orangeberry Lift

One serving of Orangeberry Lift provides 71 milligrams of vitamin C—more than 100 percent of the recommended Daily Value. And because it's made with blueberries, this drink can help slow aging and prevent cancer too.

½ cup blueberries
½ cup orange juice
2 tablespoons low-fat or skim milk or soy milk
½ cup sparkling water or seltzer

Combine the blueberries, orange juice and milk in the blender. Purée. Pour into a glass. Add the sparkling water or seltzer and stir. Serve.

**yield:**
1 serving (1½ cups)

**per serving with low-fat milk:**
152 calories, 3 g protein, 36 g carbohydrates, 1 g fat, 2 mg cholesterol, 2 g dietary fiber, 27 mg sodium. High in vitamin C and folate. A good source of carbohydrates, dietary fiber, vitamin A, thiamine, vitamin E, and potassium.

# Fresh Mint Tinkle

I found a recipe for Fresh Mint Tinkle in a carton of my mother's old recipes. It appeared in an article about "good tasting cold drinks" in the magazine *American Weekly* on July 1, 1951. I modified the recipe but kept its oh-so-1950s name. My version is good tasting *and* good for you, with 65 percent of the recommended Daily Value of vitamin C.

> ½ cup water
> ½ cup granulated sugar
> 20 mint leaves, chopped
> ½ cup fresh lime juice
> 1¼ cups red grapefruit juice
> 2 cups seltzer or sparkling water
> ice

Start by making a sweet mint syrup. Combine the water and sugar in a pot and heat until simmering. Simmer for about 5 minutes or until all the sugar has dissolved. Add the chopped mint and let steep for 10 minutes or until cool. Strain the syrup, then combine it with the lime juice and grapefruit juice in a large pitcher. Add the seltzer and stir. Serve over ice.

The mint syrup can also be refrigerated and used to prepare one serving at a time. For one glass of Fresh Mint Tinkle, combine ¼ cup of mint syrup with 2 tablespoons of lime juice, 5 tablespoons of grapefruit juice, ½ cup of seltzer. Serve over ice.

Note that because the tart juices used here require extra sweetener, the mint syrup in this recipe contains more sugar than does the mint syrup that appears in the Staples section of this book (page 178).

**yield:**
4 servings (1 cup each)

**per serving:**
136 calories, 1 g protein, 35 g carbohydrates, 0 g fat, 0 cholesterol, 0.3 g dietary fiber, 149 mg sodium. High in vitamin C.

# Persimmon Pineapple Pleasure

I love the astringent taste of persimmon. Combined with the tropical pineapple juice, it makes a delicious and nutrient-rich, high-fiber cocktail. Look for Japanese persimmon, which are sweeter and larger than the American varieties.

For a Creamy Persimmon Pineapple Pleasure omit the sparkling water and add ¼ cup plain nonfat yogurt and ½ skim milk.

> 1 large, ripe persimmon
> ½ cup pineapple juice, canned or fresh
> ½ cup sparkling water

Wash the persimmon well and remove the stem. Cut the fruit into eighths and place in blender. Add the pineapple juice and purée. Pour into a large glass. Add the sparkling water and stir. Serve plain or with ice.

**yield:**
1 serving (1 cup)

**per serving:**
188 calories, 1 g protein, 49 g carbohydrates, 0.4 g fat, 0 cholesterol, 6 g dietary fiber, 4 mg sodium. High in dietary fiber, vitamin A, vitamin C, and folate. A good source of thiamine, vitamin $B_6$, vitamin E, copper, magnesium, and potassium.

**per serving with yogurt and milk (1¼ cup):**
265 calories, 9 g protein, 59 g carbohydrates, 6 g dietary fiber, 1 g fat, 3 mg cholesterol, 113 mg sodium. High in vitamin A, riboflavin, vitamin $B_{12}$, vitamin C, vitamin D, dietary fiber, folate, calcium, magnesium and potassium. A good source of protein, thiamine, vitamin E, copper, selenium and zinc.

# persimmon

Fall is the season for persimmon, a fruit with tomato-like color and skin that is grown in Japan, China, Florida, and southern France. Wash the fruit well to clean the skin, which is edible, and enjoy persimmon raw or cooked. A ripe persimmon will feel like a ripe tomato; it will yield slightly when light finger pressure is applied to its surface.

# Papaya Zinger

This sparkling, tropical drink delivers 225 percent of the recommended Daily Value for vitamin C. Use coconut extract for that familiar island flavor without additional calories or fat.

> 1/2 papaya, peeled, seeded, and puréed or ⅔ cup fresh
>     or bottled papaya purée
> ⅓ cup orange juice
> ⅓ cup sparkling water
> fructose to taste
> few drops coconut extract
> ice
> mint leaf and slice of fresh coconut (for garnish)

Combine the papaya purée, orange juice, and coconut extract. Stir well. Add the sparkling water and stir again. Serve over ice, with a garnish of mint leave and fresh coconut wedge.

**yield:**
1 serving (1⅓ cup)

**per serving:**
96 calories, 2 g protein, 23 g carbohydrates, 0.4 g fat, 0 cholesterol, 3 g dietary fiber, 6 mg sodium. High in vitamin C, vitamin E, and folate. A good source of dietary fiber, vitamin A, thiamine, and potassium.

# Leanne's Orange Passion

My daughter Leanne lived and worked in the Dominican Republic and Mexico, where she learned to love the native fruits. Together we developed this immune-system boosting drink. Leanne suggests using champagne instead of sparkling water.

½ passion fruit
3 tablespoons orange juice
1 tablespoon frozen vanilla yogurt
1 package or ¾ teaspoon fructose (or sugar or other preferred sweetener)
½ cup sparkling water or seltzer
ice

Combine the passion fruit, orange juice, and vanilla frozen yogurt in a blender and process until smooth. Pour into a tall glass. Add the fructose and stir. Add the sparkling water or seltzer. Stir and serve over ice.

**yield:**
1 serving (¾ cup)

**per serving:**
61 calories, 2 g protein, 13 g carbohydrates, 1 g fat, 6 mg cholesterol, 1 g dietary fiber, 11 mg sodium. High in vitamin C.

# passion fruit

Passion fruit has a thick, tough skin that is purple when ripe. Cut one in half to reveal a fleshy, golden-colored mass scattered with tiny black seeds. The flesh can be used in fruit salads and, of course, in beverage recipes like this one. The seeds are edible, too; strain them out or let them fall to the bottom of your glass.

drink to your health

# 5

Vegetables make hot soups and broths excellent sources of nutrients and dietary fiber. The soups in this chapter are designed to be puréed and sipped from a mug or thermos. Many make perfect meals-on-the-go (and soothing, healthful snacks for those stuck home in bed).

# soups, broths, and hot beverages

# Creamy Shiitake Broth

**Easy to prepare** in the microwave and low in calories and fat, this hot broth carries a lot of nutritional weight. Garlic and mushrooms, particularly shiitake, enhance the immune system and may have cancer-fighting properties. Garlic also contains allicin, a natural antibiotic. And, thanks to the vegetables, miso, and soy milk, this broth is loaded with phytochemicals. Serve it immediately or purée before serving.

> ¾ cup water
> ⅓ cup chopped shiitake mushrooms (no stems)
> ⅓ cup chopped white mushrooms
> 1 teaspoon chopped white or red onion
> ½ clove garlic, minced
> 1 teaspoon red miso paste
> 2 tablespoons soy milk

Combine all the ingredients except the miso and soy milk in a microwave-safe glass measure or bowl. Microwave at high power for 2½ minutes, stirring once about halfway through cooking. Cool slightly (the broth will be very hot when it comes out of the microwave), add the miso and soy milk, then pour into blender and purée. (If you use finely chopped vegetables, you may find you can easily drink this soup without puréeing it.)

**yield:**
   1 serving

**per serving (1¼ cups):**
   50 calories, 4 g protein, 7 g carbohydrates, 1 g fat, 0 cholesterol, 1 g dietary fiber, 234 mg sodium. A good source of vitamin $B_{12}$, vitamin D, niacin, riboflavin, and pantothenic acid.

# Tomato Veggie Powerhouse

**Although preparing it** requires a little effort, you can't beat the healing power of the Tomato Veggie Powerhouse. The tomato base is high in lycopene, the antioxidant that helps prevent prostate and other cancers. Vegetables provide fiber, minerals, and loads of healthy phyotochemicals. Experiment by adding your favorite vegetables.

1 tablespoon olive oil
1 clove garlic, minced
½ cup chopped onions
1 cup chopped carrots
3 cups water
4 cups shredded cabbage or bok choy
3–4 pounds tomatoes, peeled and chopped
1 turnip, cubed
2 cups canned white or Michigan beans
1 cup dry macaroni
1 cup frozen mixed vegetables
1 teaspoon basil leaves
1 teaspoon thyme leaves
¼ teaspoon black pepper
3 teaspoons red miso paste
2½ cups fortified soy milk
3 tablespoons chopped fresh parsley

Heat the oil in a large soup pot. Add the garlic, onions, and carrots, and sauté until the onions are softened. Add the cabbage, tomato, turnip, canned beans, dry macaroni, frozen vegetables, basil, thyme, and black pepper. Cook covered for 15 minutes or until the macaroni and turnip are tender. Combine the miso and the soy milk, add to the soup and heat through. Serve topped with fresh chopped parsley.

**drink to your health**

**yield:**

10 servings (2 cups each)

**per serving:**

216 calories, 11 g protein, 38 g carbohydrate, 4 g fat, 0 mg cholesterol, 6 g dietary fiber, 145 mg sodium. High in protein, dietary fiber, vitamin A, vitamin $B_6$, vitamin $B_{12}$, vitamin C, vitamin E, folate, iron, lycopene, magnesium, thiamine, and potassium. A good source of carbohydrates, calcium, copper, niacin, riboflavin, selenium, and zinc.

# quick tomato veggie powerhouse

If you're in a real hurry, try the fast-food version of the Tomato Veggie Powerhouse: open a can of ready-to-eat, low-sodium tomato vegetable soup, microwave it in a safe container, then purée it and drink it down. The homemade version has a fresher taste, less sodium, and the added benefits of soy, but canned soup will do in a pinch.

# Savory Almond Vegetable Soup

Serve this savory soup hot or cold, as an appetizer or a midmorning or midafternoon pick-me-up. It's a great drink for blood pressure control and for healing—almonds contain phytochemicals and monounsaturated fat that can strengthen your immune system. You can also mix the chopped almonds and wheat germ and use them as a topping. This soup is based on a recipe from the Almond Board of California.

$\frac{1}{4}$ cup almonds
1 tablespoon olive oil
1 onion, chopped
$\frac{1}{2}$ cup chopped celery
$\frac{1}{2}$ sweet green pepper, chopped
4 garlic cloves, minced
4 cups fat-free chicken broth
1 tomato, chopped
$\frac{1}{2}$ cup medium white wine
1 teaspoon dried basil or 1 tablespoon fresh
$\frac{1}{2}$ teaspoon dried oregano or 2 teaspoons fresh
$\frac{1}{8}$ teaspoon black pepper
$\frac{3}{4}$ cup fortified soy milk
4 teaspoons wheat germ

Toast the almonds in a heavy saucepan. Add toasted almonds to the blender and process until they are finely chopped.

Heat the olive oil in a saucepan. Add the onion, celery, green pepper, and garlic, and sauté until tender (about 5 minutes). Add the chicken broth, tomato, wine, basil, oregano and pepper. Heat. Finally, add the soy milk and wheat germ and heat through.

Pour the soup into the blender, add the toasted almonds, and purée until smooth. Serve.

**yield:**

6 servings (1¼ cups each)

**per serving:**

132 calories, 8 g protein, 8 g carbohydrates, 6 g fat, 0 cholesterol, 2 g dietary fiber, 140 mg sodium. High in vitamin C and vitamin E. A good source of protein, vitamin A, calcium, folate, iron, magnesium, and potassium.

# Homemade Beet Borscht

Borscht, a beet soup of Russian heritage, is traditionally served hot or cold with sour cream, but yogurt makes a healthy substitute. Blackstrap molasses adds flavor and is an excellent source of iron. With bits of shredded beets, this soup is a good source of fiber. For a smoother beverage, strain the soup before serving, or purée the cooked beets rather than shredding them.

> $2\frac{1}{2}$ pounds whole red beets
> 1 quart water
> 1 large onion, quartered
> 2 bay leaves
> $\frac{1}{4}$ cup lemon juice
> $3\frac{1}{2}$ tablespoons blackstrap molasses
> 4 cups chopped tomatoes
> 6 tablespoons plain yogurt or low-fat sour cream (optional)
> brown sugar to taste (optional)

Clean and wash the beets, then place them with the water in a large pot. Bring to a boil, then cover, lower heat, and cook about 45 minutes or until the beets are tender. Remove the beets from the pot and save the liquid.

Measure the beet-cooking liquid and add enough water to make 6 cups. Peel and shred or finely chop the beets. Add the shredded beets into the cooking liquid with the onion, bay leaves, lemon juice and blackstrap molasses.

Bring the liquid to a boil, lower heat, cover and cook for 20 minutes. Remove the onion and bay leaves. Add brown sugar for sweetness if desired. Serve warm, or chill and serve cold with yogurt or sour cream.

**yield:**

6–8 servings (1½ cups each)

**per serving:**

99 calories, 3 g protein, 23 g carbohydrates, 1 g fat, 0 cholesterol, 4 g dietary fiber, 117 mg sodium. High in vitamin C, folate, iron, magnesium, and potassium. A good source of dietary fiber, vitamin A, vitamin B$_6$, calcium, and copper.

# Apple Parsnip Power

**Sweet and savory** Apple Parsnip Power is so delicious you won't believe it's healthy, too. Flavonoids (from the apples and apple juice) and folate (from the parsnips) together provide protection from arteriosclerosis. Nutrient-dense and high in fiber, two cups of this soup make a fine meal.

2 teaspoons canola oil
½ medium onion, chopped
1½ cups fat-free chicken broth
¼ teaspoon ground coriander
⅛ teaspoon cardamom
1 large apple, peeled and chunked (½ pound)
2 parsnips, peeled and chunked (½ pound)
½ cup apple juice
2 tablespoons plain nonfat yogurt

Heat the oil in a small pot, add the chopped onion and sauté for a few minutes until the onion softens. Add the chicken broth, coriander, and cardamom and bring to a boil. Then add the apple and parsnip and when the mixture is boiling again, lower the heat to simmer, cover and cook for 20 minutes until the parsnips are tender. Cool slightly. Pour the mixture into a blender and purée. Add the apple juice to thin the soup to the preferred consistency. Add a tablespoon of yogurt before serving.

**yield:**
2 servings (1 cup each)

**per serving:**
250 calories, 8 g protein, 45 g carbohydrates, 5 g fat, 0.3 mg cholesterol, 7 g dietary fiber, 154 mg sodium. High in dietary fiber, vitamin C, folate, and potassium. A good source of protein, carbohydrates, vitamin $B_6$, calcium, copper, iron, niacin, thiamine, magnesium, and phosphorus.

# Mug o' Barley

Try this quick and easy hot drink for breakfast. It's high in soluble fiber, so it helps keep cholesterol down and can help prevent diverticulosis. You'll find barley flakes (a precooked, dried and flattened form of barley) in health food stores, or look for "quick barley" near the oatmeal in your supermarket. If you have more time to cook, use pearled barley in this recipe—you'll double its dietary fiber content.

1 cup water (or 1½ cups if using pearled barley)
¼ cup barley flakes (or ¼ cup pearled barley)
lemon wedge
½ teaspoon sugar or to taste
Milk to taste

Combine the 1 cup of water, the barley flakes and the lemon wedge in a small saucepan. Bring to a boil, lower the heat and simmer for 8 minutes. (For pearled barley, use 1½ cup of water and simmer for 30 minutes or until tender.) Remove the lemon wedge. Combine the barley and liquid in a blender and purée until smooth. Pour into a mug. Add sugar or milk to taste.

**yield:**
   1 serving (1 cup)

**per serving:**
   91 calories, 3 g protein, 23 g carbohydrates, 1 g fat, 0 cholesterol, 4 g dietary fiber, 7 mg sodium. A good source of dietary fiber.

# Pumpkin Apple Healer

**Delicious in autumn** or any time of year, this creamy orange soup is high in healing vitamin A and beta-carotene. It's an excellent choice for those with fibromyalgia because it contains both malic acid (in the apple juice) and magnesium (in the pumpkin).

1 teaspoon olive oil

⅓ cup chopped onions

2 cups puréed or canned pumpkin (15 oz. can)

1½ cups apple cider or apple juice

½ cup fat-free chicken broth

½ teaspoon minced ginger

¼ teaspoon cinnamon

½ cup silken tofu or soy milk

¼ cup low-fat sour cream or yogurt (optional) for garnish

Heat the oil in a saucepan. Add the chopped onions and sauté for 10 minutes until softened. Add the pumpkin, apple juice, chicken broth, ginger and cinnamon. Simmer for about 10 minutes. Cool slightly and combine in blender with the tofu or soy milk. Purée. Serve warm with a dollop of sour cream or yogurt. Can also be served cold.

**yield:**
   4 servings (1 cup each)

**per serving:**
   121 calories, 4 g protein, 23 g carbohydrates, 3 g fat, 0 cholesterol, 4 g dietary fiber, 32 mg sodium. High in vitamin A. A good source of vitamin C, copper, iron, magnesium, and potassium.

# fresh
## pumpkin purée

To make fresh pumpkin purée, cut a pumpkin in half and remove the seeds and fibers. Place the halves cut-side down on a baking sheet and bake in a 400° oven until tender, about 40 minutes. Cool slightly, then remove the skin and cut the pumpkin into chunks. Use a food processor or blender to purée.

If you have a microwave, you can place the pumpkin half cut-side down on a microwave-safe plate or pie plate. Use a fork to pierce the skin a few times, and microwave on high for 4 minutes to soften the skin, which can then be easily removed. Let stand 3 minutes. Remove skin. Cut into cubes. Place in microwave safe container, cover and microwave on HIGH 4–5 minutes, then purée.

The pumpkin can be boiled to soften for puréeing. Cut the pumpkin in half; remove the seeds and stringy part. Cube the pumpkin with the skin on. Place in a pot with water to cover. Bring the water to a boil, lower the heat, cover, and cook until tender, about 15–30 minutes. Peel and purée.

# Hot Garlic, Carrot, and Broccoli Soup

Here's a full-flavored, savory soup that will boost your immune system—another great choice for a cold, flu, or sore throat. Garlic and onion have antibacterial properties, and cayenne or hot sauce will relieve congestion and clear the sinuses.

1 tablespoon olive oil
1 medium onion, chopped
4 cloves garlic, minced
1 carrot, peeled and sliced
2 cups chicken stock, chicken broth, or Jewish Penicillin (see page 140)
4 cups washed, peeled and cut broccoli
1 tomato, chopped
2 tablespoons chopped parsley
4 ounces spinach or kale, washed
dash black pepper and cayenne pepper
hot sauce (optional)

Heat the olive oil in a large pot. Add the onion, carrot and garlic, and sauté for 5 to 10 minutes or until the onions are tender. Add the chicken stock, broccoli, kale (if you are using it), tomato, and parsley. Bring to a boil then lower heat, cover, and cook for 15 to 20 minutes or until the broccoli is tender. Add the spinach. Continue to cook uncovered for 2 minutes. Allow to cool, then purée. Pour the soup back into the pot and stir in the black pepper and cayenne pepper. Serve. Pass the hot sauce.

**yield:**
4–6 servings ($1\frac{1}{2}$ cups each)

109 calories, 7 g protein, 13 g carbohydrates, 4 g fat, 0 cholesterol, 5 g dietary fiber, 149 mg sodium. High in vitamin C, vitamin A, and folate. A good source of protein, dietary fiber, vitamin B$_6$, vitamin E, calcium, iron, magnesium, niacin, riboflavin, and potassium.

# Tomato Pumpkin Soup

Topped with a dollop of nonfat or light yogurt or sour cream and some chopped parsley, this delicious soup is a splendid beginning to a festive fall meal. Pumpkins are high in beta-carotene and fiber; they also contain iron, vitamin C and complex carbohydrates. And, of course, they add glorious color.

> 1 tablespoon olive oil
> 1 medium onion, finely chopped
> 1 stalk celery, finely chopped
> 1 carrot, finely chopped
> 1½ cups canned or puréed pumpkin (see p. 135)
> 1 (14.5 ounce) can stewed no salt added tomatoes
> 2 cups water
> 1 teaspoon sugar
> ¼ teaspoon ground nutmeg
> black pepper to taste
> ¼ cup nonfat plain yogurt (for garnish)
> 2 tablespoons chopped parsley (for garnish)

Heat the oil in a 2–quart pot or saucepan. Add the onion, celery and carrot and sauté for 10 minutes or until softened. Add the pumpkin, tomatoes and water. Bring to a boil, lower heat, cover and cook for 10–15 minutes or until flavors blend. Remove half of the soup and transfer it to a blender or food processor. Purée until smooth. Remove and purée the other half. Pour the soup back into the pot. Add the sugar and ground nutmeg. Reheat for about five minutes and add pepper to taste. Serve in flat bowls. Garnish with a dollop of yogurt and some chopped parsley.

**yield:**

6 servings (1 cup each)

**per serving:**

83 calories, 2 g protein, 14 g carbohydrates, 3 g fat, 0 cholesterol, 4 g dietary fiber, 31 mg sodium. High in vitamin A and vitamin C. A good source of vitamin E, folate, and iron.

# Jewish Penicillin

Jewish mothers have long recognized the healing powers of hot chicken soup. The garlic and cayenne pepper in this recipe add extra healing power and help relieve congestion. Use the entire onion, including its peel, for a lovely, golden-colored broth. Add cayenne pepper or hot sauce, whatever makes you sweat!

Jewish Penicillin can be used in any recipe that calls for chicken stock. You can also freeze one-cup portions and use them for emergencies. Quickly thaw the individual portions in a pot or in the microwave and add frozen vegetables, cooked rice, or pasta.

> 4 pounds raw chicken (wings or legs are fine)
> 12 cups water
> 1 onion, quartered and unpeeled
> 12 sprigs parsley
> 2 stalks celery, cut into $\frac{3}{4}$-inch lengths
> 4 carrots, scrubbed and cut into $\frac{3}{4}$-inch lengths
> 2 bay leaves
> 3 cloves garlic, sliced
> $\frac{1}{4}$ teaspoon black pepper, cayenne pepper, or hot sauce

In a large soup pot, add the chicken and water and bring to a boil. Skim off the surface froth. Lower heat and add the onion, parsley, celery, carrots and bay leaves. Cover and cook for about an hour. Remove from heat. Allow to cool slightly. Strain and add pepper, cayenne pepper, or hot sauce to taste.

If desired, refrigerate stock and remove fat then reheat before serving.

**yield:**

8 servings (1 cup each)

**per cup (estimated):**

179 calories, 26 mg protein, 6 g carbohydrates, 5 g fat, 81 mg cholesterol, 0 g fiber, 106 mg sodium. High in protein, vitamin A, and
zinc. A good source of potassium.

# quick chicken stock

No time to prepare chicken stock? Ask your local deli
or Asian restaurant if they would sell you a quart or
two. If you're using canned chicken broth or soup,
check to make sure the first ingredient on the label is
chicken or chicken broth. And look for a brand that is
low in sodium—less than 500 mg per serving.

# Manhattan Clam Chowder

This tomato and clam chowder is hearty and healthful. Clams provide vitamin $B_{12}$, copper, and healthy omega-3 fatty acids, while tomatoes and potatoes deliver immune-enhancing glutathione. Onions and garlic add an extra immune system boost. You'll need a spoon for this one.

1 tablespoon olive oil
½ cup chopped onion
½ cup chopped celery
2 cloves garlic, minced or sliced
2 cups cubed potato
1 (10 oz.) can clams with liquid or 1 pint fresh clams
     and liquid
½ cup water
2–3 tablespoons chopped fresh parsley
1 teaspoon dried thyme
2 cups chopped peeled and seeded tomatoes
dash sugar and ground black pepper

Heat the oil in a medium pot. Add the onion, celery, and garlic and sauté for about 5 minutes or until softened. Drain the liquid from the clams (about ¾ cup) and add it to the pot along with the water, reserving the clams for later use. Bring to a boil. Add the potatoes, 2 tablespoons of the parsley, and thyme and cook over medium heat until the potatoes are tender, about 8 minutes. Add the reserved clams (or fresh clams and liquid) and the tomatoes and heat through. Finally, add the sugar, pepper, additional parsley, and water if necessary. Serve.

**yield:**

4–6 servings (about 1 cup each)

**per serving:**

131 calories, 3 g protein, 23 g carbohydrates, 4 g fat, 2 mg cholesterol, 3 g dietary fiber, 180 mg sodium. High in vitamin $B_{12}$, vitamin C, and copper. A good source of dietary fiber, vitamin A, vitamin $B_6$, magnesium, potassium, and thiamine.

# Creamy Split Pea Soup

**Thick and creamy,** this soup is high in protein and very high in fiber, with 16 grams per serving. If that's too much fiber for you, try thinning the soup with chicken or vegetable broth. You'll get a delicious vegetarian soup if you use vegetable stock (see staples section) instead of water and omit the chicken.

> 7 cups water, or 7 cups vegetable stock for vegetarian soup
> 1 pound chicken legs (4 drumsticks), skin removed (omit for vegetarian version)
> 1 cup chopped carrots
> 1 cup chopped onions
> 3 cup split peas
> 1 clove garlic, minced
> ½ teaspoon oregano
> ¼ teaspoon thyme
> dash pepper

Combine the water and chicken in a large soup pot. Bring to a boil and skim the foam. Lower the heat and add the remaining ingredients. Cover and cook for 45 minutes. Remove the chicken. Purée the remaining soup in batches in a blender or food processor.

**yield:**
8 servings (1 cup each)

**per serving:**
270 calories, 22 g protein, 42 g carbohydrates, 2 g fat, 20 mg cholesterol, 16 g dietary fiber, 34 mg sodium. High in protein, dietary fiber, vitamin A, folate, magnesium, potassium, and zinc. A good source of carbohydrate, copper, iron, selenium.

# Phyto-Favorite

Served hot or cold, the Phyto-Favorite will boost your immune system. The garlic, onions, watercress, and tomato contain lots of healing phytochemicals. Drink it hot if you're suffering from a cold or flu.

1½ teaspoons olive oil
1 clove garlic, minced
1 cup chopped onions
2 cups fat-free chicken broth
2 tablespoons short-grain white rice
1 bunch watercress, about 4 cups
½ cup plain skim yogurt
2 tablespoons chopped tomato (for garnish)

Heat the oil in a pot. Add the garlic and onions and sauté on low for about 10 minutes until the onions are softened. Add the chicken broth and white rice and bring to a boil. Lower the heat, cover and cook for 15 minutes. Meanwhile, wash and drain the watercress, remove the thicker stems, and coarsely chop the remaining watercress.

Add the watercress and continue to cook for 5 more minutes. Combine all the ingredients in a blender and purée. Then add the yogurt and purée again. Serve immediately or chill. Garnish with chopped tomato.

**yield:**
4 servings (¾ cup each)

**per serving:**
92 calories, 7 g protein, 12 g carbohydrates, 2 g fat, 0.6 mg cholesterol, 1.4 g dietary fiber, 124 mg sodium. High in vitamin A, vitamin C, and beta-carotene. A good source of protein, calcium, and potassium.

# My Best Gazpacho

Gazpacho is a spicy, cold Spanish soup made with chopped summer vegetables. My version is healthy and without added oil, and with avocado for added protein, monounsaturated oils, and potassium. Of course, with all the vegetables, it's high in fiber and packed with phytochemicals, too.

> 1 large tomato, quartered
> ¼ cup cubed avocado
> 2 tablespoons chopped green onion
> 2 tablespoons chopped sweet green pepper
> 1 teaspoon Worcestershire sauce
> dash salt and pepper
> dash hot sauce

Combine the ingredients in the blender and purée. More hot pepper sauce can be added for taste.

**yield:**
1 serving (1 cup)

**per serving:**
111 calories, 3 g protein, 14 g carbohydrates, 6 g fat, 0 cholesterol, 5 g dietary fiber, 78 mg sodium. High in vitamin A, vitamin C, and potassium. A good source of dietary fiber, vitamin $B_6$, copper, folate, niacin, iron, magnesium, and thiamine.

# Oyster Stew

Canned oysters make this stew quick and easy. Check labels and buy oysters with the lowest sodium content you can find (Geisha brand, from Korea, is one). Alternatively, you can prepare this with fresh oysters. In a quick low fat and low calorie soup, oysters provide iron, omega-3 fatty acids, vitamin $B_{12}$ and zinc.

1 teaspoon olive oil
2 tablespoons finely chopped onion
2 tablespoons finely chopped celery, including leaves
1 can (8 ounces) whole oysters
1 cup 2-percent-fat milk or soy milk
1/4 teaspoon Worcestershire sauce

Heat the olive oil in a small pot. Add the onion and celery and sauté until softened, 5 or more minutes. Combine the liquid from the oyster can, the milk, and the Worcestershire sauce in the pan and heat slowly. Cut the oysters into bite size pieces and add to the pot. Continue to heat about 2 or 3 minutes until hot. Serve.

To prepare with fresh oysters, use about a dozen fresh oysters, reserving the liquid. When the onions and celery are softened, add the oysters and sauté until the edges are curling and slightly darkened, and then add the remaining ingredients and enough reserved liquid to make it the consistency you prefer.

**yield:**
2 servings (1 cup each)

**per serving:**
160 calories, 12 g protein, 11 g carbohydrates, 7 g fat, 3 g mono-fat, 2 g saturated fat, 71 mg cholesterol, 0.3 g dietary fiber, 197 mg sodium. High in protein, vitamin $B_{12}$, vitamin D, copper, iron, calcium, magnesium, riboflavin, selenium, and zinc. Good source of vitamin A, vitamin C, thiamine, and potassium.

# Souper Miso

Although it's made from soy, which can help protect our bodies from heart disease and cancer and relieve the symptoms of menopause, miso is very high in sodium. A cup of Souper Miso can be so calming, however, that I've decided to include it here. Try it when you need to relax, or between meals for a caffeine-free beverage.

1 cup boiling water, slightly cooled
1 teaspoon red miso paste or red soy paste
Tiny cubes of firm tofu (for garnish)

Combine the water and miso paste and stir until the miso is dissolved. Drink while hot, garnished with tiny tofu cubes.

**yield:**
1 serving (1 cup)

**per serving:**
10 calories, 1 g protein, 1 g carbohydrate, 0 fat, 0 cholesterol, 0.2 g dietary fiber, 214 mg sodium.

6

The drinks in this chapter, made with low-fat or nonfat dairy, soy, or rice milks, make wonderful snacks or dessert beverages. Frothy or smooth, milks are generally easy on the digestive system. Fruit and vegetable juices add flavor and nutritional benefits.

# Orange Creamsicle Shake

This creamy shake will remind you of the popular orange-vanilla ice cream treats you enjoyed as a kid. Packed with nutrients and high in calories, fiber, protein, and carbohydrates, it makes an excellent breakfast substitute. Cut the recipe in half if you'd prefer a lower-calorie beverage.

1½ cups nonfat vanilla frozen yogurt, low-fat, or regular

½ cup 1 percent milk (or your choice)

1 banana, cut into thick slices

3 tablespoons frozen orange juice concentrate

2 teaspoons dry egg-white powder

Combine all ingredients in a blender and purée.

**yield:**
1 serving (1⅓ cups)

**per serving with nonfat frozen yogurt and 1 percent milk:**
564 calories, 20 g protein, 118 g carbohydrate, 2 g fat, 8 mg cholesterol, 3 g dietary fiber, 335 mg sodium. High in protein, carbohydrates, vitamin $B_6$, vitamin C, folate, calcium, potassium. A good source of dietary fiber, vitamin A, thiamine, riboflavin, vitamin D, copper, iron, magnesium, and selenium.

# Calming Almond Milk

In the Ayurvedic healing tradition of India, a glass of warm almond milk is believed to lower anxiety. This high-protein, low-carbohydrate drink is also a good source of vitamin D and calcium, which help prevent osteoporosis and build strong bones. The calcium, magnesium, and potassium are good for lowering blood pressure. You can strain this milk if you like, but you'll be losing the benefits of the fiber and some of the nutrients.

2 tablespoons whole almonds
1 cup low-fat or reduced fat or whole milk

Soak the almonds in water (just enough to cover them) overnight. Strain and remove the skins, then purée or finely chop the almonds in a blender. Warm the milk, add it to the blender, and purée. Serve warm.

**yield:**
1 cup

**per serving (with low-fat milk):**
219 calories, 13 g protein, 16g carbohydrates, 12 g fat, 1.5 g saturated fat, 15 mg cholesterol, 2.3 g dietary fiber, 130 mg sodium. High in protein, vitamin D, and calcium. A good source of dietary fiber, vitamin A, magnesium, and potassium.

# Tang-Tang

Cranberry and pineapple juices provide vitamin C, healing phytochemicals, and lots of tangy taste to this dairy-free drink. Double or triple the recipe and store Tang-Tang in the refrigerator so it's ready when you are. Use the Rice Cure recipe (see page 156) for homemade rice milk (store-bought works fine, too), or substitute yogurt for the rice milk if you're so inclined.

> $\frac{1}{3}$ cup cranberry juice cocktail
> $\frac{1}{3}$ cup pineapple juice
> $\frac{1}{4}$ cup rice milk

Combine the ingredients in a glass. Stir. Add ice and serve.

**yield:**
   1 serving (about 1 cup)

**per serving (with rice milk):**
   119 calories, 0.3 g protein, 30 g carbohydrates, 0.2 g fat, 0 cholesterol, 0.3 g dietary fiber, 4 mg sodium. High in vitamin C.

# Orange Froth

This frothy drink is an excellent source of isoflavones (from the soy) and limonenes (from the citrus), both of which help prevent cancer. The orange juice also provides the antioxidant vitamin C, which promotes a healthy immune system.

Dried egg white adds protein and creates froth, but this drink is delicious without the egg white if it's not available. (Never use fresh raw egg whites, which can carry dangerous bacteria, in this or other beverages. For information on dried egg white, see page 215).

$3/4$ cup freshly squeezed orange juice
$1/2$ cup soy milk or vanilla-flavored fortified soy milk
1 teaspoon dried egg white
$1/2$ teaspoon vanilla extract (optional, not needed if vanilla-flavored soy milk is used)
ice

Combine ingredients in a blender process until frothy. Serve over ice.

**yield:**
1 serving

**per serving with fortified vanilla-flavored soy milk:**
167 calories, 6 g protein, 31 g carbohydrates, 2 g fat, 0 cholesterol, 0.4 g dietary fiber, 75 mg sodium. High in vitamin A, vitamin $B_{12}$, vitamin C, and a good source of protein, carbohydrates, thiamine, vitamin E, folate, calcium, magnesium, and potassium.

# Raspberry Rumble

Dairy milk can help lower cholesterol and blood pressure, especially in men. Lower cholesterol levels reduce the risk of heart disease, as do the fiber and vitamin C in this sweet pink drink.

> ½ cup fresh or frozen unsweetened raspberries
> ½ cup 1 percent milk or soy milk
> ¼ teaspoon sugar (optional)

Combine the ingredients in a blender and process until smooth. The sugar is optional but does sweeten the milk nicely. Strain the milk before drinking it if you don't like all those raspberry seeds.

**yield:**
1 serving (1 cup)

**per serving (unstrained) with 1 percent milk:**
81 calories, 5 g protein, 13 g carbohydrates, 2 g fat, 5 mg cholesterol, 4 g dietary fiber, 62 mg sodium. High in dietary fiber, riboflavin, vitamin $B_{12}$, vitamin C, vitamin D, and calcium. A good source of vitamin A, folate, magnesium, manganese, and phosphorus.

# New-Fashioned
# Vanilla Milk Shake

Old-fashioned milk shakes are laden with fat. This smooth, "new-fashioned" shake, made with nonfat and low-fat dairy products, is a wonderful, much healthier substitute. It's high in carbohydrates, protein, and calcium—a great choice for any time of the day. Go ahead and treat yourself.

> 1½ cups nonfat frozen vanilla yogurt
> ½ cup skim milk

Combine ingredients in a milkshake machine or blender. Blend and serve.

**yield:**
1 serving (about 1⅓ cups)

**per serving:**
343 calories, 13 g protein, 69 g carbohydrate, 0.2 g fat, 2 mg cholesterol, 0 dietary fiber, 273 mg sodium. High in carbohydrate, calcium, protein. A good source of riboflavin, vitamin D, and iron.

# The Rice Cure

Bland and easy to digest, rice is often recommended for stomach problems and when recovering from diarrhea. The Rice Cure recipe comes from the folk medicine tradition. Mild rice milk is also a good source of folate, one of the vitamins that helps restore balance in the intestinal tract. Try the Rice Cure on its own or use it in place of commercial rice milk in any of the recipes in this book.

    2 cups water
    ¼ cup rice
    a drop or two of vanilla extract
    1 teaspoon honey or to taste
    dash cinnamon

Bring the water to boil in a pot. Add the rice, cover and simmer for twenty minutes. Add the vanilla extract and honey. Sprinkle with cinnamon. Strain and drink the liquid.

**yield:**
  2 servings (1 cup each)

**per serving with rice (included):**
  108 calories, 2 g protein, 24 g carbohydrates, 0.2 g fat, 0 cholesterol, 0.2 g dietary fiber, 7 mg sodium. A good source of folate.

# cinnamon

In homeopathic, Asian, and folk medicine traditions, cinnamon is used to help stop diarrhea. Cinnamon is also said to help bronchitis, colds, cough, fever, indigestion, sore throat, and infection, and it may actually have the power to destroy bacteria. In a Kansas State University study, researchers found that when cinnamon was added to apple juice, the bacteria levels in the juice decreased.

# Mildred's
# Banana Rice Healer

**My mother used** to say that bananas, apples, tea, and chocolate could help overcome diarrhea. I used banana and chocolate in this recipe, along with rice milk, which is easy on the digestive system. Bananas also supply potassium, an important mineral that can be depleted after a bout of diarrhea. For an apple-carob rice healer, substitute carob rice milk for the chocolate rice milk and applesauce for the banana.

> 1 cup chocolate-flavored rice milk (or 1 cup plain rice
>     milk plus 2–3 teaspoons chocolate syrup)
> 1 medium banana
> dash salt
> 2 teaspoons honey or other sweetener (optional)

Combine the milk and banana in a blender and process until smooth. Stir in the salt. Add honey or sweetener if desired. Serve.

**yield:**
   1 serving (about 1⅓ cups)

**per serving:**
   312 calories, 2 g protein, 73 g carbohydrate, 3 g fat, 0 cholesterol, 5 g dietary fiber, 250 mg sodium. High in vitamin $B_6$, and vitamin C. A good source of vitamin E, potassium, and sodium.

# Apple Ambush

The pectin in the carob and applesauce in this drink helps stop diarrhea. Carob also contains vegetable tannins, which help restore balance in the digestive tract. Don't forget that dash of salt; diarrhea can deplete your body's sodium supply.

> 1 cup carob rice milk (or 1 cup rice milk plus 1 to 2 teaspoons carob powder)
> ½ cup unsweetened, natural applesauce
> dash salt

Combine the carob rice milk and applesauce and stir until smooth. Add the salt. Serve.

**yield:**
   1 serving (1½ cups)

**per serving:**
   203 calories, 1 g protein, 46g carbohydrates, 3 g fat, 0 cholesterol, 2 g dietary fiber, 242 mg sodium.

# Vanilla Mellow

Mild rice milk is easy to digest, while yogurt with active cultures helps restore healthy bacteria in the intestines after diarrhea or other digestive difficulties. Vanilla Mellow is high in carbohydrates, so it's calming, too. Try it before bedtime.

2 cups water
¼ cup white rice
2 tablespoons plain skim yogurt
dash vanilla extract
1 teaspoon honey or other sweetener
cinnamon (for garnish)

Bring the water to a boil. Add the rice, lower the heat to simmer, then cover and cook for 20 minutes. Strain the mixture, or leave it unstrained and eat the rice, too. Pour the liquid in a mug; stir in the yogurt, vanilla, and honey. Sprinkle with cinnamon and serve hot or cold.

**yield:**
2 servings (1 cup each)

**per serving (with rice):**
117 calories, 3 g protein, 26g carbohydrates, 0.2 g fat, 0.3 mg cholesterol, 0.2 g dietary fiber, 19 mg sodium. A good source of folate.

# Ultimate Egg Nog

This low-calorie version of the holiday favorite is a healthy beverage choice at any time of the year. It's high in protein and calcium, which help build strong bones and muscles. Egg substitutes are pasteurized, so they're safe to drink right out of the container. Fresh raw eggs should not be used because they can carry salmonella bacteria.

> ½ cup skim milk
> 1 teaspoon sugar
> ½ teaspoon vanilla extract
> ½ cup egg substitute
> nutmeg (as garnish)

Combine the milk, sugar, vanilla extract, and egg substitute in a blender. Process just until foamy and well combined. Pour in a glass or mug, sprinkle with nutmeg, and serve cold.

**yield:**
  1 serving (1 cup)

**per serving:**
  125 calories, 16 g protein, 12 g carbohydrates, 0.2 g fat, 2 mg cholesterol, 0 dietary fiber, 263 mg sodium. High in protein and calcium. A good source of vitamin A, riboflavin, vitamin D, iron, and potassium.

# Mango Milk

Luscious mangoes are loaded with phytochemicals, antioxidants, and beta carotene, making this sweet milk drink nutritious as well as delicious. Because it contains magnesium and calcium, Mango Milk may also help prevent insomnia.

> ½ fresh mango
> 1 cup soy milk
> 1 teaspoon sunflower seeds

Combine the ingredients in a blender and purée.

**yield:**
1 serving (1½ cups)

**per serving:**
214 calories, 11 g protein, 31 g carbohydrates, 6g fat, 0 mg cholesterol, 2 g dietary fiber, 107 mg sodium. High in calcium, magnesium, protein, vitamin A, vitamin $B_{12}$, vitamin C, and vitamin E. A good source of vitamin $B_6$, carbohydrates, folate, thiamine, vitamin D, pantothenic acid, iron, and potassium.

# Blueberry Vision

During World War I, British flyers noticed that when they ate bilberry jam before flying at night, their night vision seemed to improve. Today experts know that bilberries and their cousins blueberries, cranberries, and blackberries, contain anthocyanosides, antioxidants that strengthen the capillaries in the retina. Anthocyanosides are also thought to be helpful in preventing age-related eye problems such as cataracts and macular degeneration.

> 1 cup vanilla-flavored fortified soy milk
> 1 cup blueberries, fresh or frozen
> dash cinnamon

Combine the soy milk and the blueberries in the blender and purée. Serve with a dash of cinnamon.

**yield:**
1 serving ($1\frac{1}{3}$ cups)

**per serving:**
231 calories, 7 g protein, 43 g carbohydrates, 4 g fat, 0 cholesterol, 4 g dietary fiber, 99 mg sodium. High in vitamin A, vitamin $B_{12}$, vitamin C, vitamin E, and calcium. A good source of protein, carbohydrates, dietary fiber, thiamine, vitamin D, folate, magnesium, and potassium.

# Meno-Magic

**Temper the symptoms** of menopause with this nutrient-dense drink. I also call this "Quick Breakfast in a Glass"—it makes a healthy, well-balanced breakfast for those on the go.

> 1 cup chocolate-flavored soy milk (or one cup plain soy
>     milk plus 1 or 2 teaspoons of chocolate syrup)
> ½ cup orange juice
> 1 tablespoon oat bran or wheat germ

Combine the ingredients in a large glass and whisk together.

**yield:**
    1 serving (1½ cups)

**per serving with oat bran:**
    279 calories, 9 g protein, 52 g carbohydrates, 5 g fat, 0 cholesterol, 1 g dietary fiber, 40 mg isoflavones. High in vitamin C, vitamin D, folate, calcium, copper, and magnesium. A good source of protein, carbohydrates, iron, and potassium.

**per serving with toasted wheat germ:**
    291 calories, 10 g protein, 51 g carbohydrates, 6g fat, 0 cholesterol, 1 g dietary fiber, 40 mg isoflavones. High in protein, vitamin C, vitamin D, folate, calcium, copper, and magnesium. A good source of carbohydrates, iron, potassium, and zinc.

# soy and isoflavones

Soy contains healthy isoflavones, daidzein and genistein, that may prevent heart disease and certain cancers. But when some soy foods (including soy hot dogs and soy burgers) are processed, isoflavones can be removed. Check food labels so you can be sure of a product's isoflavone content.

Studies indicate that soy protein will help lower cholesterol. To be effective, 30–50 mg per serving of isoflavones and 6.25 grams of soy protein are needed four times a day to lower cholesterol. A serving of soy that provides 30–50 mg isoflavones and 6.25 g soy protein are:

$\frac{1}{2}$ cup cooked green soybeans

$\frac{1}{2}$ cup cooked soy beans

$\frac{1}{4}$ cup roasted soy butter

$\frac{1}{4}$ cup roasted soy nuts

$\frac{1}{2}$ cup soy flour

$\frac{1}{4}$ cup soy grits

$\frac{1}{2}$ cup firm tofu

1 cup soy milk

$\frac{1}{2}$ cup cooked TVP (textured vegetable protein)

$\frac{1}{2}$ cup tempeh

# Strawberry Slider

Kids will love the Strawberry Slider's creamy pink color and fruity taste, and it's so much more nutritious than the watered-down juice drinks that are popular today. It makes a great snack for adults, too: high in nutrients, low in fat and calories.

8 strawberries
2 tablespoons orange juice
⅔ cup vanilla-flavored fortified soy milk or 1 percent milk
Dash sugar (optional)

Combine the ingredients in a blender and process until smooth. Serve.

**yield:**
1 serving (1 cup)

**per serving with vanilla-flavored fortified soy milk:**
142 calories, 5 g protein, 25 g carbohydrates, 2.4 g fat, 0 cholesterol, 2 g dietary fiber, 61 mg sodium. High in vitamin A, vitamin $B_{12}$, vitamin C, vitamin E, folate. A good source of protein, dietary fiber, thiamine, vitamin D, pantothenic acid, calcium, magnesium, and potassium.

# Cucumber Cooler

Smooth, cool Cucumber Cooler, made with vegetables and lowfat dairy products, provides 249 milligrams of calcium—25 percent of the recommended Daily Value—for strong, healthy bones. Onion and garlic contribute phytochemicals to keep your immune system purring.

1 cucumber, peeled
½ cup skim or low-fat buttermilk
1 teaspoon chopped onion
1 clove garlic, minced
2 tablespoons plain nonfat yogurt
½ teaspoon chopped fresh chives

Cut peeled cucumber into chunks and place in a blender. Add the buttermilk, onion, garlic and yogurt and process. Pour into tall glass. Top with chopped chives. Serve.

**yield:**
1 cup

**per 1 cup serving:**
106 calories, 8 g protein, 17 g carbohydrates, 2 g fat, 5 mg cholesterol, 2 g dietary fiber, 158 mg sodium. High in calcium, potassium, and a good source of protein, vitamin C, folate, and magnesium.

# New Belly Bliss

A healthy belly is a blissful belly. The live cultures in this yogurt-based drink will help heal the digestive tract. Ginger, in addition to adding its distinctive flavor, will soothe your stomach and may help prevent ulcers.

½ cup non-fat plain yogurt
½ cup water
⅛ teaspoon grated fresh ginger

Combine the ingredients in a glass and whisk to combine. Serve.

**yield:**
1 serving (1 cup)

**per serving:**
69 calories, 7 g protein, 10 g carbohydrate, 0.2 g fat, 2 mg cholesterol, 0 dietary fiber, 97 mg sodium. High in calcium. A good source of protein, riboflavin, and vitamin $B_{12}$.

# The Peacemaker

When stress has got you down, turn to the Peacemaker. This creamy drink provides the key nutrients for stress relief: carbohydrates and vitamin $B_6$. And it's healthy in other ways, too. Bananas supply potassium, and prunes and raisins are packed with anti-aging, immune-system-boosting antioxidants.

½ cup apple juice
½ cup red grape juice
4 pitted dried prunes
¼ cup raisins
2 whole cloves
2 whole allspice
½ banana
1 cup 1 percent milk
½ cup plain nonfat yogurt

In a pot, combine juices, prunes, raisins, cloves and allspice. Bring to a boil. Lower heat and cook for 5 minutes. Remove from heat. Allow to set until cool. Remove the cloves and allspice. Add the banana and purée the mixture. Pour back into pot. Add the milk and yogurt and stir to combine. Serve warm or chill.

**yield:**
2 servings (1 cup each)

**per serving:**
281 calories, 9 g protein, 60 g carbohydrates, 2 g fat, 6 mg cholesterol, 3 g dietary fiber, 118 mg sodium. High in carbohydrates, riboflavin, vitamin $B_6$, vitamin C, calcium, and potassium. A good source of protein, dietary fiber, vitamin A, thiamine, vitamin $B_{12}$, vitamin D, pantothenic acid, copper and magnesium.

The recipes in this chapter
are those you'll use again
and again (and in other
recipes in this book). The
concentrated sugar, mint,
and fruit syrups can be
used to sweeten any num-
ber of hot or cold bever-
ages, while super-nutritious
vegetable broth serves as
the perfect base for a variety of soups. You'll find the
other "basics" included
here to be equally adapt-
able.

# Watermelon Ice Cubes

Watermelon cubes make a wonderful addition to iced tea, selzer water, and other drinks. As they melt, they add flavor and nutrition. Try making ice cubes using other fruits, too.

3 cups cubed watermelon

Remove the seeds from the watermelon and purée in a blender or processor. Pour into ice cube trays and freeze. Store ice cubes in sealed plastic freezer bags and use as needed.

**yield:**
1 tray or 14–16 cubes

**per cube:**
10 calories, 0.2 g protein, 2 g carbohydrates, 0.1 g fat, 0 cholesterol, 0.2 g dietary fiber, 0.7 mg sodium.

## migraine relief

For migraine headache relief, try sucking on a watermelon ice cube. Ice can prevent blood vessels from dilating painfully. The watermelon cubes provide a bit of sugar, which may also be helpful (low blood sugar can sometimes trigger migraines).

# Cough Syrup

This recipe is a modified version of one I found in a collection of folk remedies called "Mountain Makin's in the Smokies," published in 1957 by the Great Smoky Mountains Natural History Association. According to the book, Mrs. Stanley Cooley learned to make cough syrup from her mother, who used it when her children had colds.

    4 ounces (¾ cup) flaxseed
    1½ cups water
    ½ cup sugar
    juice of 3 lemons
    4 tablespoons honey

Add the flaxseed to a small saucepan filled with 1½ cups water. Bring to a boil then lower heat to simmer. Cook until the liquid has boiled down to half its original amount. Remove from heat and stir in the sugar, lemon juice, and honey. Cool. Store in the refrigerator for up to one week or freeze. Give a spoonful as needed for coughs or sore throat.

**yield:**
  1 cup

**per tablespoon:**
  83 calories, 1 g protein, 15 g carbohydrates, 2 g fat, 0 cholesterol, 2 g dietary fiber, 4 mg sodium.

# Sugar Syrup

Use this simple sugar syrup to sweeten iced beverages. It will blend with your drink instantly, without leaving a pile of undissolved sugar at the bottom of your glass.

½ cup water
1 cup granulated sugar

Pour water into a pot and stir in sugar. Bring to a boil, stirring occasionally. To prevent a messy boil-over, keep your eye on the pot. As soon as you see the mixture boil, lower the heat to simmer. Simmer, stirring occasionally, for 5 minutes. Cool. Store in a jar in the refrigerator and use as needed.

**yield:**
1 cup

**per teaspoon:**
48 calories, 13g carbohydrates, 0 protein, 0 fat, 0 cholesterol, 0 dietary fiber, 0.4 mg sodium.

# Ginger Syrup

This delicious syrup is used as a base for Homemade Ginger Ale (see page 114). You can also use a tablespoon or two to sweeten and flavor other drinks.

1 ounce chopped ginger (about 2 tablespoons)
1 cup water
1 tablespoon granulated sugar

In a small pot, combine the ginger, water, and sugar. Bring to a boil, then lower the heat and simmer, uncovered, for 10 minutes. Strain. Store in the refrigerator.

This recipe can be doubled or tripled depending on your needs.

**yield:**
1 cup

**per tablespoon:**
4 calories, 0 protein, 1 g carbohydrate, 0 fat, 0 cholesterol, 0 dietary fiber, 1 mg sodium.

# Ginger Juice and Hot Ginger Tea

Ginger juice adds the delicious snap of ginger to hot and cold teas and other beverages (try adding it to cranberry or pineapple juice). You can make fresh ginger juice by cutting a piece of ginger into thin slices, then pressing the slices through a garlic press. Or use a ginger grater that can be purchased in Asian markets. Press grated ginger through a sieve to extract the juice.

Use ginger juice to make this relaxing tea, which will soothe the stomach and can help prevent motion sickness.

> 1 teaspoon grated or minced ginger root or 1 teaspoon
>    ginger juice
> 1 cup boiling water

Combine the grated or minced ginger root or ginger juice with boiling water and steep for 5 minutes. Strain if necessary. Serve and sip.

**yield:**
  1 serving (1 cup)

**per serving:**
  1 calorie, 0 protein, 0.3g carbohydrate, 0 fat, 0 cholesterol, 0 dietary fiber, 7 mg sodium.

# Mint Syrup

Homemade mint syrup adds sweetness and flavor to cold drinks or hot teas.

1 cup water
½ cup granulated sugar
10–12 fresh mint sprigs, chopped

Combine the water and sugar in a pot and bring to a boil. Simmer until the sugar is dissolved, about 5 minutes. Add the mint. Remove from heat and allow to cool. Strain. Store in a jar in the refrigerator and use as needed.

**yield:**
1 cup

**per tablespoon:**
24 calories, 6g carbohydrate, 0 fat, 0 fiber, 0 cholesterol, 0 dietary fiber, 0.5 mg sodium.

# Sun Tea

Sun tea, simple to make and filled with healthy flavonoids, is clear and less bitter than tea made with boiling water. Try flavoring with added juices: mango, peach, orange, or lemon.

> 2 quarts cold water
> 5 tea bags or 3–5 tablespoons loose green or black tea
> ice

Combine water and tea or tea bags in a glass container. Cover and place in the sun for 3 to 5 hours. Remove the bags or strain the tea; refrigerate. Serve cold with ice.

**yield:**
8 servings (1 cup each)

**per serving:**
2 calories, 0 protein, 1 g carbohydrate, 0 fat, 0 cholesterol, 0 dietary fiber, 7 mg sodium.

# Refrigerator Tea

You CAN make iced tea in the refrigerator, you'll just need to use more tea than usual—cold water does not draw flavor from the tea as well as hot water does.

> 1 quart cold water
> 5 tea bags or 3–5 tablespoons loose tea
> ice

Combine ingredients in a glass pitcher or jar. Cover. Refrigerate for 8 or more hours. Remove bags or strain. Serve over ice.

**yield:**
4 servings (1 cup each)

**per serving:**
0 calories, 0 protein, 0 carbohydrate, 0 fat, 0 cholesterol, 0 dietary fiber, 7 mg sodium.

# fruit syrups

When you buy a fruit-flavored soft drink, you're usually getting more sugar (in the form of high fructose corn syrup) than you bargained for. You can prepare fruit drinks at home and get more real fruit taste using these easy-to-make fruit syrups. For a light, delicious drink, mix 2 or 3 tablespoons of your favorite homemade syrup into a glass of water or seltzer, add ice (and extra sweetener if necessary), and enjoy. Fruit syrups can also add flavor to any cold drink or hot beverage.

# Blackberry Syrup

Only three ingredients are needed to make your own Blackberry Syrup from fresh or frozen blackberries. Use 2–3 tablespoons of this Blackberry Syrup in the Blackberry Sparkle recipe in the Cocktails or Other Sparkling Beverages section or use it to add flavor and sweetness to your favorite beverage. Raspberries can be used in place of the blackberries.

> 2 cups granulated sugar
> 1 cup water
> 2¼ cups fresh blackberries or a 12 oz. package frozen unsweetened blackberries

Stir the sugar and water together in a pot. Heat slowly to boiling, stirring occasionally. As soon as the mixture begins to boil, lower heat and simmer for 5 minutes. Add the berries, stir and simmer for another 10 minutes. Cool and strain. A thin, clear liquid will result. To remove more of the pulp from the berries, mash the berries through a sieve or cheese cloth lined strainer with a wooden spoon. Or a Foley food mill can also be used to remove most of the seeds from the berries.

Store in a sealed jar in the refrigerator. Mix 2 or 3 tablespoons with plain seltzer or water, or use to sweeten and flavor any drink.

**yield:**
2¼ cups

**per 2 tablespoons:**
98 calories, 0.2 g protein, 25 g carbohydrates, 0 fat, 0 cholesterol, 1 g dietary fiber, 1 mg sodium.

# Cranberry Syrup

This syrup does contain sugar, which helps temper the tartness of the berries. Use it in place of the blackberry syrup in the recipe for Blackberry Sparkle and you'll have a Cranberry Sparkle.

  2 cups granulated sugar
  1 cup water
  12-oz package fresh cranberries

Stir the sugar and water together in a pot. Heat slowly to boiling, stirring occasionally. As soon as the mixture begins to boil, lower heat and simmer for 5 minutes. Add rinsed cranberries and simmer another 10 minutes. Cool and strain using a Foley food mill (some pulp and tiny seeds will remain) or press the berries, using a wooden spoon, through a cheesecloth lined strainer. If you would like a rich and clear red liquid, just allow the cranberry syrup to drip though a cheesecloth. Cool and refrigerate in a glass jar. Mix 2 or 3 tablespoons with plain seltzer or water, or use to sweeten any drink.

**yield:**
  2¼ cups

**per 2 tablespoons:**
  95 calories, 0 protein, 25 g carbohydrates, 0 fat, 0 cholesterol, 0.8 g dietary fiber, 1 mg sodium.

# Unsweetened Blueberry Syrup

**Instead of adding** the sugar to the blueberries immediately, this syrup is made without sugar and then a sugar of your choice can be added. Flavor seltzer or your favorite beverage with 2–3 tablespoons of blueberry syrup and then add the sweetener of your choice to taste. Two to 3 teaspoons of granulated sugar, the sugar syrup in the Staples section, or ginger or mint syrup would work.

In a large glass, add 2–3 tablespoons of the blueberry syrup, 2–3 teaspoons of sugar, mint or ginger syrup, or 1–2 packages or ¾ teaspoon of Splenda or any non-caloric sweetener, fill the glass with water or seltzer, stir and add ice.

> 1 cup water
> 2¼ cups fresh blueberries or 12 oz. frozen unsweetened blueberries

Combine the blueberries and water in a pot. Bring to a boil and simmer for 10 minutes. Cool and press through a Foley Food Mill, a cheesecloth lined strainer, or a sieve. Store in a sealed jar in the refrigerator and use within a week or two.

**yield:**
  1½ cups

**per 2 tablespoons:**
  15 calories, 0.1 g protein, 4 g carbohydrates, 0.2 g fat, 0 mg cholesterol, 1 g dietary fiber, 1mg sodium.

**drink to your health**

# Unsweetened Raspberry Syrup

Add unsweetened raspberry syrup and your favorite sweetener (caloric or noncaloric) to seltzer or the beverage of your choice. Delicious!

    1 cup water
    1½ cup fresh raspberries or 12 oz. frozen unsweetened
        raspberries
    8 packages Splenda non-caloric sweetener (6 teaspoons)

Wash the fresh raspberries if using those. Add the raspberries and the water to a pot. Bring the mixture to a boil, lower the heat and simmer for 10 minutes. Cool slightly. Press through a sieve or Foley food mill. You will have about 1¼ cup. To this stir in 8 packets or 2 teaspoons of Splenda or a sweetener of your choice. A packet of Splenda (¼ teaspoon) is equal to the sweetening power of 2 teaspoons of sugar. Store in a sealed jar in the refrigerator and use within a week or two.

**yield:**
  1¼ cups

**per 2 tablespoon:**
  17 calories, 0.3 g protein, 4 g carbohydrates, 0.2 g fat, 0 mg cholesterol, 1 mg sodium.

# Vegetable Broth

Use this low-sodium vegetable broth as a base in soup recipes. It's also delicious enough to enjoy plain or with cooked rice, millet, barley or other grains for added fiber.

Shiitake mushrooms make this broth a nutritional knock-out. They're high in B vitamins and contain immune system strengthening phytochemicals and cholesterol-lowering eritadenine. If you can't find fresh shiitake, substitute maiitake, enoki, or oyster mushrooms. White button mushrooms can also be used; they'll provide good flavor and B vitamins but contain few phytochemicals.

> 2 teaspoons olive oil
> 2 cups chopped shallots or onions
> 3 garlic cloves, minced
> 2 cups chopped celery
> 2 cups chopped carrots
> 3½ oz. fresh shiitake mushrooms, chopped
> ¼ cup chopped fresh parsley
> 2 bay leaves
> 1 teaspoon dried thyme
> 3 quarts water

Heat the olive oil in a soup pot. Add the shallots or onions, garlic, celery, carrots, and mushrooms. Sauté for several minutes until the onions are softened. Add the parsley, bay leaves, thyme, and water. Bring to a boil, then lower the heat to a simmer. Cover and cook for 1½ hours. Cool and strain. Use immediately or freeze in 1 or 2 cup quantities for use in future recipes.

**drink to your health**

**yield:**

8 servings (2 quarts)

**per cup:**

79 calories, 2 g protein, 11 g carbohydrates, 4 g fat, 0 cholesterol, 0 dietary fiber, 52 mg sodium. High in vitamin A. A good source of vitamin $B_6$ and folate.

Who knew improving your vitality and immunity could be this delicious? Whether you want to slow down the effects of aging, relieve arthritis or a headache, lower your cholesterol levels, help to prevent heart disease or overcome insomnia, or get over a cold or the flu, you can drink to your health. Use the ailments index to identify those drinks that are best-suited to help you address your particular condition.

# anti-aging

To lengthen your life, help fight the affects of aging, and prevent age-related diseases like cancer and heart disease, choose foods that are high in antioxidants: vitamins C and E, selenium, carotenoids (including beta-carotene), monounsaturated fats, and healing phytochemicals. Blueberries and cranberries are particularly noted for their anti-aging properties.

### recommended for fighting the effects of aging:
Mike's Blueberry Egg Cream
Mango Sunrise
Ginger Mango Super Smoothie
Orange Julia
Soy Peach Blueberry Perk-Up
Tomato Veggie Powerhouse

# appetite loss/
# low body weight

To gain weight, you need to increase your caloric intake. But not just any calories will do. To ensure healthy weight gain, eat foods that provide calories and nutrition. If you're too busy to stop for a full meal, drink a nutrient-dense beverage on the run.

Brewer's yeast, an excellent source of B vitamins, can act as an appetite stimulant, as can the following herbs: caraway, cardamom, chamomile, chicory, cinnamon, coriander, dill, fenugreek, ginger, lemon balm, peppermint, rosemary, sage, and turmeric.

### recommended for healthy weight gain:
Purple Protein Power Shake
Lemon Balm Anxiety Reducer
Nutrient Dense Pear Avacado Abundance
Ginger Apricot Support
Morning Superstart
Soy Peach Blueberry Perk-Up

# arteriosclerosis

To prevent arteriosclerosis, or hardening of the arteries, keep your cholesterol level low and choose foods that are low in fat and high in soluble fiber. Keep intake of saturated fats (animal and dairy fats such as meat, milk and cheese) and trans- or hydrogenated fats (vegetable shortening and margarine) to a minimum.

Certain nutrients, including the antioxidants, can also help lower cholesterol levels. The plant chemicals such as quercetin, which is found in apples, onions, and black tea, can lower cholesterol, and resveratrol, found in red wine and Concord grapes, may also be helpful. Garlic has blood-thinning properties. To help lower homocysteine levels, which causes blood vessel damage, increase the folate in your diet.

### recommended for the prevention of arteriosclerosis:

Orange Ginger Thirst Quencher

Sun Tea and Refrigerator Tea

Grape Tea

Papaya Zinger

High-C

Ginger Apricot Support

Apple Parsnip Power

Blackberry Wine Cooler

# anemia

General weakness, loss of appetite, dizziness, inability to concentrate, headache, and apathy can be signs of iron-deficiency anemia, or lack of iron in the blood. Most common in pregnant women and persons with chronic illnesses, iron-deficiency anemia can be detected with a simple blood test performed by your doctor.

To prevent or reverse iron-deficiency anemia, eat foods that are rich in iron (leafy green vegetables, fish, and black-strap molasses) and the B vitamins.

**recommended for the prevention of iron-deficiency anemia:**

Tomato Cocktail

Homemade Beet Borscht

Tomato Veggie Powerhouse

Oyster Stew

# arthritis

Because rheumatoid arthritis is an autoimmune disease, foods that strengthen the immune system—fruits, vegetables, whole grains—can help patients with the condition. Antioxidants can strengthen the immune system and help slow joint deterioration. Choose foods that are rich in beta carotene (spinach and other dark leafy vegetables, apricots and other yellow or deep orange vegetables) and vitamin C (especially cantaloupe, broccoli, strawberries, peppers and cranberry juice). In the folk medicine tradition, cherries are a remedy for arthritis.

High-fat diets can make arthritis worse, so avoid saturated fats such as those found in meats and dairy products. Some patients may notice that their pain or arthritic discomfort increases when they eat certain foods, particularly wheat products, dairy products, corn, citrus, and eggs. Talk to your doctor, and keep a food diary to see how certain foods affect your body. Try eliminating vegetables in the nightshade family—tomatoes, white potatoes, peppers, and eggplant—from your diet.

Some people believe that wearing a copper bracelet offers arthritis relief, so eating foods that are rich in copper (whole grains, leafy green vegetables, almonds and other nuts) might be beneficial. Ginger and turmeric, herbs with anti-inflammatory properties, may also help.

## recommended for the relief of arthritic symptoms:

Arthritis Relief

Piquant Pomegranate

Apple Ambush

Blackberry Sparkle

Creamy Split Pea Soup

Melon Mango Invigorator

Oyster Stew

Hot Ginger Tea

Green Ginger Tea

# athletic injuries

Maintain a healthy, well-balanced diet when your body is healing from an athletic injury. Complex carbohydrates will help maintain muscle strength, while vitamin E can help prevent muscle soreness. And magnesium will keep muscles flexible so that injury can be avoided. Drink plenty of water to help prevent muscle spasms and cramps.

To help heal broken or fractured bones, eat a diet rich in the B vitamins, zinc, calcium, vitamin D, and protein.

## recommended for those with athletic injuries:

One-Two Punch

Caribbean Powerhouse

Melon Mango Invigorator

Morning Superstart

Purple Protein Power Shake

Hi-Pro

# bladder or
# urinary tract infections

Bacterial infections in the bladder or urethra are particularly common in women. If you have a bladder or urinary tract infection, try drinking a glass of water every hour for eight hours to dilute the urine and help flush out bacteria. Cranberry and blueberry juice can also help eliminate unwanted bacteria from the bladder and urinary tract.

**recommended for prevention and relief of bladder or urinary tract infections:**

UTI Cocktail

Good Time Party Punch

Unsweetened Blueberry Syrup

Cranberry Fizz

Tummy Rescue Remedy

Mike's Blueberry Egg Cream

# cancer

Experts believe that diet can play a crucial role in reducing the risk of cancer, particularly cancer of the breast, bowel, and prostate. Eating the recommended five servings of fruits and vegetables each day may reduce the rate of some cancers by more than 20 percent.

In October 1998, the American Institute for Cancer Research released their International Report on Cancer Prevention. Among their recommendations for cancer prevention:

- Eat a plant-based diet, one that is rich in a variety of vegetables, fruits, legumes, and minimally processed foods.
- Maintain a healthy weight. Limit weight gain during adulthood to less than 11 pounds.
- Eat five or more servings a day of a variety of fruits and vegetables.
- Eat seven or more servings a day of a variety of grains, legumes, and roots.
- Limit consumption of refined sugar.
- Avoid alcoholic beverages, or limit yourself to no more than two each day (no more than one a day for women).
- Limit fatty and salty foods. Choose modest amounts of appropriate vegetable oils.
- Avoid eating charred foods. Consume grilled or broiled meat and fish or cured and smoked meats only occasionally.

**recommended for cancer prevention:**

Cancer Phyter

High-C

Melon-Mango Invigorator

Mango Milk with Green Tea

Orange Froth

Creamy Split Pea Soup

My Best Gazpacho

Phyto Favorite

Hot Garlic, Carrot and Broccoli Soup

## cholesterol

Heart disease, the leading cause of illness and death in the United States, is related to high blood pressure and high blood cholesterol. A cholesterol level of 200 or lower is recommended.

A healthy diet that is low in cholesterol, fat, trans- and saturated fat will help reduce blood cholesterol. Eat plenty of fruits, vegetables, and whole grains. Soluble fiber—found in oats, rice, barley, and dried beans—can also help lower blood cholesterol levels.

**recommended for lowering cholesterol:**

Mug o' Barley

Mildred's Banana Rice Healer

Sy's Lime Rickey

Raspberry Rumble

## chronic fatigue syndrome

Foods that are high in protein, fiber, vitamins, and magnesium can help the fatigue associated with Chronic Fatigue Syndrome. Try a high-fiber, high-protein drink in the morning or as a snack for an energy boost.

Allergies and food sensitivities can also contribute to Chronic Fatigue Syndrome. While allergies usually last a lifetime, food sensitivities can change with time and are usually associated with food groups, such as citrus fruits or milk products. Try changing the foods you eat and see how you feel. The most common food allergies involve corn, eggs, milk, sugar, and wheat.

Some experts believe chronic fatigue syndrome may be related to a low blood pressure syndrome called Neurally Mediated Hypotension. A moderate salt intake and higher liquid consumption can be helpful for persons with Neurally Mediated Hypotension and may therefore benefit those with Chronic Fatigue Syndrome as well.

### recommended for those with chronic fatigue syndrome:

Soy Peach Blueberry Perk-Up
Soy Peach Strawberry Smoothie
Avocado Smoothie
Hi-Pro
Tomato Veggie Powerhouse
Creamy Split Pea Soup

# colds and bronchitis

A cure for the common cold has eluded scientists for decades. But research is continuing to prove that herbs and nutrients can help prevent and shorten the duration of colds and respiratory infections like bronchitis. Hot drinks are also comforting for cold sufferers; they help get the mucous flowing and raise the body temperature, stimulating the immune system to increase its production of infection fighting antibodies.

To prevent a cold or to help heal one, try increasing your intake of one or more of the nutrients listed here:

**Vitamin C,** abundant in tropical and citrus fruits, boosts the immune system to help fight off infections.

### drinks high in vitamin C include:
Good Time Party Punch
High C
Elizabeth's Healing Cocktail
Lemon Aid
Raspberry Lemon Aid
Leanne's Orange Passion

**Echinacea,** long used by Native Americans to treat a variety of conditions, seems to support the immune system by increasing the production and activity of white blood cells. Try taking echinacea when you have a cold or a sore throat. If used for longer than 6 to 8 weeks for cold prevention, echinacea's beneficial effects can diminish.

Talk to your doctor before using echinacea if you have lupus, tuberculosis, or multiple sclerosis, or if you are allergic to flowers in the daisy family. And don't take echinacea if you're taking corticosteroids (like Decadron, prednisone) or Cyclosporine (Neoral, Sandimmune).

### drinks containing echinacea include:
Echinacea Tea with Lemon and Honey
Aromatic Astragalus Tea

**Zinc** strengthens the immune system and may help shorten the duration of a cold.

### drinks high in zinc include:
Tomato Veggie Powerhouse
Jewish Penicillin Chicken Stock
Creamy Split Pea Soup
Oyster Stew

**Cayenne and other hot peppers** act as expectorants and decongestants.

**drinks that contain cayenne and other hot peppers include:**

Hot Garlic, Carrot and Broccoli Soup

Jewish Penicillin

**Hot beverages** act as decongestants and soothers.

**hot beverages include:**

Phyto-favorite

Creamy Shitake Broth

Licorice Root Soother

Hot Garlic, Carrot and Broccoli Soup

Doubly Green Tea

Jewish Penicillin

# cold sores

Foods high in lysine, such as corn, kidney beans, and split peas, can help relieve and prevent cold sores, which are caused by the Herpes Simplex virus. Avoid citrus and other acid foods, which can be painful and irritating, and avoid nuts, chocolate, and seeds. These latter contain the amino acid that is food for the virus. Smooth cream soups and milkshakes can be soothing.

**recommended for soothing cold sores:**

Creamy Split Pea Soup

New-Fashioned Vanilla Milkshake

# constipation

To keep bowel movements regular and prevent constipation, drink plenty of water (six to eight glasses a day) and make sure you're eating enough fiber. Twenty-five to thirty-five grams of dietary fiber per day are recommended. If you're not used to eating that much fiber, increase your daily intake slowly. High fiber foods include vegetables, especially peas, beans, and broccoli; bran cereals and wheat bran; oat bran; whole grains; and fruits, particularly dried fruits such as raisins, figs, and prunes. You can also add fiber to your diet using a fiber supplement such as psyllium or powdered flaxseed.

Other foods and beverages that can help relieve constipation include coffee, perhaps because the caffeine stimulates the digestive system; prunes and prune juice, which contain a bowel stimulant called dihydroxyphenyl isatin; and grapes and raisins, which contain tartaric acid, a natural laxative.

**Note:** See your doctor if your constipation is accompanied by pain, fever, or blood.

### recommended for the relief of constipation:

Tutti Fruiti on the Rocks
Faux Café
Psyllium Soother
Prune Raisin Smoothie
Creamy Split Pea Soup

# diarrhea

Diarrhea can be caused by certain foods or by an infection, virus, or food poisoning. Whatever the cause, when you have diarrhea you'll need to replace lost fluids by drinking lots of water, herb and black or green teas, mineral water, flat cola beverages, diluted sports drinks, or flat ginger ale. Avoid carbonated beverages, which can cause gas and add to the discomfort. Start eating solid foods and fiber gradually as your condition improves. Pectin, found in apples and bananas, can help firm the stools. (Try applesauce rather than apple juice, which can contribute to diarrhea).

Because it involves fluid loss, diarrhea can also drain your body of vital electrolytes. Replace lost sodium by drinking bouillon, diluted sports drinks, and soy, rice, or barley miso. Bananas will help firm stools and replace lost potassium.

Folate and berry leaf teas (blackberry, blueberry, and raspberry) can help heal and soothe an irritated colon. Yogurt with live cultures helps replace good bacteria in the intestines.

The tannins in green tea also combat diarrhea; the longer the tea is steeped, the more tannins the tea will contain. The problem, however, is that green tea also contains caffeine, which can exacerbate a diarrhea problem. Try drinking decaffeinated green tea. Or, because most of the caffeine from tea is drawn into the water in the first minute of steeping, steep green tea for one minute, pour the liquid away, then use the bag again to get more tannins and less caffeine. Use discretion and moderation, and see what works best for you.

If diarrhea lasts more than a few days, see a doctor.

## recommended for treatment of diarrhea:

The Rice Cure

Mildred's Banana Rice Healer

Apple Ambush

Greenberry Tea

Souper Miso

Vanilla Mellow

## diverticulosis

Diverticula, or pouches, form in the intestines as we age. Diverticulosis is the painful condition that occurs when these pouches become inflamed and infected.

To prevent diverticulosis, eat a low-fat, high-fiber diet (20 to 25 grams of fiber daily), drink at least 8 glasses of water a day, and lower your stress level. Avoid low-fiber, processed foods such as white bread, white rice, crackers and cookies, and try to include some wheat bran in your diet. Like psyllium and flaxseed, wheat bran absorbs water in our bodies, softening the stools and adding bulk so that they can move smoothly through the intestines.

Once you have diverticulosis and the intestinal pouches are infected, however, a high-fiber diet can make the problem worse. Until the infection is over, most types of fiber should be avoided. Do not eat popcorn, celery, nuts, seeds, or seeded foods like tomatoes, cucumbers, and raspberries. So that you are not constipated during the healing process, apples, peaches, bananas, pears, oranges, seedless grapes, raisins, prunes, carrots, lettuce, bran and bran cereals, and whole wheat breads may be eaten in moderation.

## recommended for the prevention of diverticulosis:
Mug o' Barley
Watermelon Chamomile Frosty
Creamy Split Pea Soup
Psyllium Soother
Blueberry Smoothie
Pear and Blueberry Smoothie

# fibromyalgia

Fibromyalgia, often called the "baby boomers' disease," is an immune system disorder characterized by fatigue and pain in the muscles and connective tissues. At this time there is no cure for fibromyalgia but medication, exercise, and lifestyle changes have allowed patients to manage their symptoms and improve their quality of life.

Doctors recommend that patients with fibromyalgia eat a healthy diet that is low in caffeine, sugar, and fat, and high in fiber. And magnesium and malic acid have been shown to alleviate some of the symptoms. High-magnesium foods include soy and soy products, rice, bananas, dark leafy greens, avocado, blackstrap molasses, oysters, and yogurt. Malic acid is found naturally in apples and can be taken as a dietary supplement. It's also used commercially to control pH levels in processed foods; when used, it will appear on a product's list of ingredients.

## recommended for those with fibromyalgia:
Nutrient Dense Pear-Avocado Abundance
Golden Quencher
Avocado Smoothie
Vanilla Mellow
Spirit Lifting St. John's Wort Tea
Pumpkin Apple Healer

# gas and gas pains

Gas is a natural byproduct of digestion. Some foods, however, produce more gas when they are digested than others do. Beans are infamous for their gas-producing properties—their high carbohydrate content results in extra gas when digested. (Soy beans are higher in protein and are easier to digest). Milk products can cause painful gas, especially in those that are lactose-intolerant. If milk is a problem for you, try low-lactose or lactose-free varieties, acidophilus milk, rice milk, soy milk, or nut milks.

Gas is also caused when there is excess air in the stomach, which can result from eating too fast, eating foods that are beaten (such as blender drinks), drinking carbonated drinks, drinking through a straw, riding a bike with your mouth open, or chewing gum.

For gas relief and to aid in digestion, peppermint and chamomile are recommended. Anise, caraway, coriander, ginger, and turmeric can also be helpful.

## recommended to relieve gas and to aid in digestion:

Basil Tea

Soothing Spearmint Tea

Lemon Balm Anxiety Reducer

# hangover

To help relieve the pain and discomfort of a hangover, and to prevent the dehydration associated with alcohol consumption, drink plenty of liquids, especially water and those containing fructose. Found naturally in honey, tomato juice, and any fruit juice, fructose is quickly absorbed into the blood stream. It will raise your energy level and can help your body burn off alcohol. (Some experts also believe that vitamin C can help clear the body of alcohol.) Caffeine and cold drinks can help shrink blood vessels in the brain and relieve alcohol-related headaches.

**recommended for hangover relief:**

Iced Mochaccino

Sy's Lime Rickey

Quick Comeback

Kiwi Strawberry Smoothie

# headache

Stress and tension headaches are caused by tightness in the head and neck muscles. For drinks that may help relieve stress or tension headaches, see Stress.

Vascular or migraine type headaches are caused when the blood vessels in the brain dilate. Vascular headaches can be triggered by hormones, hunger, changes in altitude, changes in weather, bright or flashing lights, smoking, or food allergy.

If you suffer from migraines, avoid foods that may trigger them, including chocolate, red wine, aged cheeses, monosodium glutamate (MSG), and hot dogs. These foods contain tyramine, an amino acid that causes the blood vessels first to constrict and then to dilate, causing headache pain. Caffeine, ice water, and cold drinks can bring headache relief by helping enlarged arteries contract.

Among the nutrients believed to help prevent migraine headaches are magnesium (found in bran, wheat germ, soy, peanut butter, and yogurt); calcium and vitamin D (found in milk and enriched soy milk); and riboflavin (found in dairy foods, eggs, leafy vegetables and enriched and whole grains).

Ginger may also help prevent migraines by blocking the action of the prostaglandins that cause pain and inflammation in blood vessels. Add $\frac{1}{3}$ teaspoon of powdered ginger to your favorite beverage when you feel a migraine coming on.

**recommended for migraine relief:**

Hot Ginger Tea

Iced Mochaccino

Iced Refrigerator and Sun Tea

Soothing Spearmint Tea

Watermelon Ice Cubes

Tummy Rescue Remedy

## age-related hearing loss

Recent studies have shown that age-related hearing loss may be related to low levels of vitamin $B_{12}$ and folate in the bloodstream. Try increasing the amount of these nutrients in your daily diet.

### recommended for the prevention of age-related hearing loss:

Avocado Smoothie

Ginger Mango Smoothie

Morning Superstart

## heart disease

One of the leading causes of illness and death, heart disease is related to and can be caused by high blood pressure and high cholesterol. To protect yourself against heart disease, maintain a diet that is high in fruits, vegetables, and low-fat dairy foods, and low in sodium, saturated fat, and total fat. Oat bran and dried beans are high in soluble fiber and can help lower cholesterol levels and the risk of heart disease. The minerals potassium, magnesium, and calcium, which are often lacking in the American diet, are important in preventing high blood pressure and heart disease.

The flavonoids in red wine, green tea, and fruits and vegetables, the calcium in skim milk, the mono fat in almonds, and the omega-3 fatty acids in fish and flax can also help prevent heart disease.

(Other major factors for developing heart disease include stress, smoking, lack of exercise, and obesity. To protect your heart health, get plenty of exercise, use stress reduction techniques, maintain a normal body weight, and avoid tobacco products).

**recommended for the prevention of heart disease:**

Ginger Apricot Support

Melon-Mango Invigorator

Soy Peach Blueberry Perk-Up

Manhattan Clam Chowder

Oyster Stew

Strawberry Wine Cooler

Blackberry Wine Cooler

Good Time Party Punch

Kiwi Soy Smoothie

Mighty Blue Healer

## hemorrhoids

Fiber! The best way to prevent the pain and itching of hemorrhoids is to eat at least 25 grams of fiber every day. Foods that are high in fiber are vegetables, fruits, nuts and whole grains. Psyllium, flaxseed, bran, and wheat germ add fiber to the diet and bulk to the stool. Avoid coffee and caffeine drinks, which have diuretic properties that can contribute to hard stools.

Folate, potassium, selenium, zinc, vitamin A, vitamin C, vitamin E, and protein are recommended as healing nutrients for hemorrhoids.

**recommended for the prevention of hemorrhoids:**

Mighty Blue Healer

Creamy Split Pea Soup

Prune Raisin Smoothie

Soothing Spearmint Tea

## high blood pressure

A diet rich in fruits, vegetables and low-fat dairy foods and low in saturated fat, total fat, and sodium is recommended for persons with high blood pressure.

Garlic and onion are said to reduce high blood pressure; red wine can help lower blood pressure when used in moderation.

Minerals that may help lower or control blood pressure include calcium (found in low-fat yogurt or milk, buttermilk, and fortified soy milks) potassium, and magnesium.

## recommended to prevent or control high blood pressure:

Blackberry Wine Cooler
Nutrient-Dense Pear-Avocado Abundance
Grape Tea
Green Tea With Punch
Blueberry Smoothie
High Po

# hypoglycemia

Low blood sugar can cause weakness, hunger, nervousness, dizziness, trembling, or perspiration. Small, frequent meals that include whole grains, beans, soy products, and foods that are high in protein, complex carbohydrates, and fiber can help keep blood sugar levels even. Persons with hypoglycemia should avoid caffeine and alcohol.

Chromium, a mineral found in whole grains, brewers yeast, molasses, eggs and cheese, helps convert glucose into energy, and may also help keep blood sugar levels even.

## recommended for those with hypoglycemia:

Ultimate Egg Nog
Homemade Beet Borscht
Savory Almond Vegetable Soup
Creamy Split Pea Soup
Soy Peach Blueberry Perk-Up

# insomnia

Insomnia can be caused by stress, hunger, menopausal or post menopausal hormone shifts, or carbohydrate needs. The night can also loom long due to pain, too much caffeine, daytime naps, or inadequate exercise.

Hot, herbal, caffeine-free teas sipped slowly before bedtime can be helpful in inducing sleep and relaxation. Passion flower, lemon balm, chamomile, linden flower, skullcap, valerian, and lavender, are known for their calming effects.

**recommended for treatment of insomnia:**
Passion Flower Bedtime Tea
Grandmom Rose's Cup of Tea
My Best Gazpacho
Mango Milk
Lemon Balm Anxiety Reducer
Soothing Spearmint Tea
Calming Almond Milk

## intestinal virus (gastroenteritis or stomach flu)

Flat ginger ale, Mom's old stand-by for stomach flu, can actually help when a person has an intestinal virus; ginger helps calm an upset stomach and relieves digestive problems. Ginger or stomach-soothing mint teas can also be slowly sipped to help calm the stomach and replace lost liquids.

Fluid replacement is important when flu is accompanied by vomiting. Persons who are vomiting should sip water, tea, or mineral water until they are able to try Jell-O and bland, solid foods, such as mashed potatoes and rice.

If flu symptoms last more than 2 to three days, call your doctor.

**recommended for treatment of an intestinal virus or flu:**
Hot Ginger Tea
Tummy Rescue Remedy

## irritable bowel syndrome

Irritable Bowel Syndrome (IBS) can involve diarrhea, constipation, flatulence, or alternating diarrhea and constipation. While stress is considered a major factor in the condition,

208

depression, caffeine, laxatives, gastrointestinal illness, antibiotics, and sleep irregularity can also contribute.

A healthy diet that is low in fat and contains moderate amounts of fiber can help calm irritable bowels. (Fiber helps keep the stools soft and easy to pass, but too much fiber can cause gas and bloating). Drink at least eight glasses of water a day to help ensure regularity.

Hot, caffeine-free teas (try chamomile or lemon balm) may help sufferers of Irritable Bowel Syndrome because they are soothing.

**recommended for those with irritable bowel syndrome:**
    Soothing Spearmint Tea
    Lemon Balm Anxiety Reducer
    Mint Syrup
    Chocolate Kiwi Smoothie
    Psyllium Soother
    Licorice Root Soother

# macular degeneration

Macular degeneration, which generally occurs in persons over the age of 55, is a genetic disease that affects the retina and can lead to blindness. There is no cure for the disease once it occurs, but research suggests that zinc may help protect the eye from macular damage. Zinc-rich foods include oysters, clams, shrimp, beef and beef stock, chicken and chicken stock, yogurt, wheat germ, soy, peanut butter, and miso.

**recommended to prevent macular degeneration:**
    Oyster Stew
    Jewish Penicillin
    Blueberry Smoothie
    Pear and Blueberry Smoothie

# menopausal symptoms

Exercise and the right diet may help reduce the symptoms of menopause, which include hot flashes, insomnia, forgetfulness, loss of creativity, osteoporosis, vaginal dryness, and lessened sexual desire. The right diet should include healthy, low-fat foods and foods that contain vitamin E and fish oils.

Foods that are high in phytoestrogens replace lost estrogen naturally and can also help relieve symptoms. Try including whole wheat, flax, broccoli, cauliflower, split peas, spinach, coffee, apples, barley, carrots, cherries, chick peas, garlic, yams, and soy in your diet. Some researchers believe that just two servings of soy a day can bring results. A serving of soy would be one cup of soy milk, $\frac{1}{3}$ cup of soybeans, $\frac{1}{3}$ cup of roasted soy nuts, $\frac{1}{3}$ cup of soy flour, $\frac{1}{4}$ cup of textured vegetable protein (TVP), or $\frac{1}{4}$ cake of tofu. The herbs oregano, thyme, and turmeric may also have some estrogenic properties.

After menopause, the metabolism slows and fewer calories are needed to maintain a healthy weight, so lower calorie and nutrient-dense foods are recommended. Because hormonal changes can increase the risk for heart disease, an increase in the antioxidant vitamins would also be beneficial. And because osteoporosis is more common after menopause, extra calcium should be included in the diet. (See Osteoporosis.)

## recommended for the relief of menopausal symptoms:

Meno-Magic
Savory Almond Vegetable Soup
Soy Do It
Hot Garlic, Carrot and Broccoli Soup

# mood elevating/depression

Research suggests that a high-carbohydrate, low-protein diet can improve mood. High carbohydrate foods supply the body with tryptophan, which increases the level of the feel-good neurotransmitter serotonin in the brain.

Eating chocolate, cayenne peppers, and other hot peppers, may help, too: These foods stimulate the production of endorphins, natural tranquilizers that make a person feel calm and increase positive feelings of well-being.

S-adenosyl-L-methionine, better known as SAMe, is another substance that may affect mood-controlling neurotransmitters in the brain. SAMe is created from methionine, an amino acid or protein found in soy, beans, and meat. SAMe is now being sold as an antidepressant or supplement. However, if your body is lacking in vitamin $B_{12}$, vitamin $B_6$ or folate, the methionine in SAMe will convert to homocysteine, which is bad for the heart. If you're taking SAMe, make sure you're eating plenty of whole grains, beans, fish, poultry, and leafy green vegetables.

The herb St. John's Wort is also thought to enhance serotonin levels and relieve feelings of depression.

### recommended for mood elevation:
Chocolate Kiwi Smoothie
Spirit Lifting St. John's Wort Tea
New Fashioned Vanilla Milkshake
Purple Protein Power Shake
Cocoa Fruit Smoothie

## motion sickness

Ginger, which calms the stomach, can be used to prevent and alleviate motion sickness.

### recommended for the prevention and treatment of motion sickness:
Ginger Syrup
Homemade Ginger Ale

## osteoporosis

To prevent osteoporosis, include calcium-rich dairy products and leafy green vegetables in your diet, especially if you are female and postmenopausal. Avoid caffeine, alcohol, and foods that are high in phosphorus, including red meat and soft drinks. Foods that are high in phytoestrogens, particularly foods containing soy, can also promote bone strength.

Your body needs vitamin D to absorb calcium from the foods you eat. Foods that are rich in vitamin D include tuna, salmon, and enriched milk products. You can also get vitamin D by spending a little time in the sun—just 10 to 30 minutes a week will do the trick.

**recommended for the prevention of osteoporosis:**
Cucumber Cooler
Strawberry Slider
Caribbean Powerhouse
Soy Do It
Calming Almond Milk

## premenstrual syndrome

To reduce the symptoms of premenstrual syndrome (PMS), which include bloating, mood changes and depression, acne, headaches, fatigue, weight gain, breast tenderness, and cravings for sugary or salty foods, stick to a low-fat, high-fiber diet. Avoid foods that are high in sugar, caffeine, and sodium (which contributes to bloating).

Foods that are high in complex carbohydrates may give some relief from mood swings. Vitamin $B_6$ (a natural diuretic that can relieve bloating), vitamin E (to relieve breast tenderness), vitamin A, and the minerals magnesium and calcium are recommended.

**recommended for the prevention
or relief of PMS symptoms:**
Cocoa Fruit Smoothie
Mellow Mama
Hot Garlic, Carrot and Broccoli Soup
Mango Milk

## stomach ulcers

Abdominal pain between meals or after drinking alcohol or acidic beverages such as orange juice, coffee, tea, or colas, can signal the presence of an ulcer. If you think you have an ulcer, see your doctor, who can diagnose the source of your pain and will prescribe antibiotics if necessary (ulcers are believed to be caused by bacterial infections).

A healthy diet that is low in fat and high in fiber can help prevent ulcers. And stress does play a role: even though ulcers are caused by bacterial infections, you are more likely to develop an ulcer if you are under stress.

If you are taking antibiotics for your ulcer, your medication may be killing off "friendly" bacteria along with the harmful bacteria in your body. Yogurt with live cultures may help to restore the beneficial bacteria that antibiotics can elminate.

### recommended for the prevention of stomach ulcers:

Elizabeth's Healing Cocktail

New Belly Bliss

Island Powerhouse

Vanilla Mellow

The Rice Cure

The Peacemaker

## stress

A stress-fighting diet is centered around fruits, vegetables and whole grains. Avoid high-fat foods and limit your caffeine intake. Learn to relax with a hot cup of herbal tea in the middle of the day—chamomile and lemon balm are soothing and relaxing.

### recommended for stress reduction:

The Peacemaker

Kiwi Strawberry Smoothie

Lemon Balm Anxiety Reducer

Ginger Yogurt Support

Soothing Spearmint Tea

## varicose veins

The best way to prevent varicose veins is to keep your circulation system in tip-top shape. Drink plenty of fluids, at least 8 glasses of water each day, to promote circulation. High-vitamin and -mineral foods—vegetables, fruits, and whole grains—are excellent for keeping veins in good condition, as are antioxidants, especially vitamins C and E.

Bioflavonoids, found in citrus fruits, apricots, blueberries, blackberries, apples, onions, cherries, and green tea, help maintain vascular strength. They protect the blood vessels and reduce platelet aggregation, acting as natural blood thinners.

### recommended for the prevention of varicose veins:

Fresh Mint Tinkle

Grape Tea

Apple Parsnip Power

Pear and Blueberry Smoothie

Morning Superstart

Frosty Apricot Mint Cooler

# Resources

- Yogi brand Echinacea Tea also contains many ingredients including astragalus root, fennel, cardamom, clove, black pepper, and mint which together make a very good flavored tea. Yogi has a catalogue available by calling 1–800–359–2940 and a web site: *http://www.yogitea.com*. They are located at 2545 Prairie Road, Eugene, OR 97402.
- Just Whites, distributed by Deb-El Foods Corporation, 2 Papetti Plaza, Elizabeth, NJ 07207, are 100% fat free, all-natural powdered egg whites which contain no artificial flavoring, coloring, additives or preservatives. Requires no refrigeration. If you can't find it in your local market, call 1–800–421–EGGS and they will mail it to you.
- Alvita teas package over 100 teas. They can be found at *www.twinlab.com* (the parent company) or at *www.alvita.com*. They also package a new group of teas called Remeteas which combine herbs for remedies and they have great names like Masculinitea, Detoxitea, Resistabilitea, and Visibility.
- Marco Polo Blackberry syrup comes in a quart bottle (actually 33 ounces) and in 2 tablespoons (1 oz.) there are 105 calories. The ingredients are blackberry juice and sugar. It is a product of Slovenia imported by Adria Imports, Inc. 57–58 59th Street, Maspeth, NY 11378.

- Reed's Original Ginger Brew is an all-natural Jamaican style ginger ale, distributed by Original Beverage Corp, CA, 800–997–3337, *www.reedsgingerbrew.com*.
- The all-natural ginger ale distributed by Health Valley, Irwindale, CA 91706–7811. Ingredients: sparkling spring water, fructose, natural juices, natural flavorings of ginger root, molasses and other natural herbal extracts.
- Soy Dream brand soy milks are manufactured by Imagine Foods. They can be contacted at *www.imaginefoods.com* or at Imagine Foods, Inc., 350 Cambridge Avenue, Suite 350, Palo Alto, CA 94306, 650–327–1444, FAX 650–327–1459.
- For various herbal and non-herbal teas, contact The Republic of Tea, The Minister of Supply (020), Post Office Box 1589, Novato, California 94948–1589 or call 1–800–298–4TEA to receive a catalogue.
- Splenda is a low-calorie sweetener, made from sugar and tastes like sugar. Does not break down when heated so it can be used in baking. There are no warning labels required on foods that contain Splenda. According to the manufacturer "it passes through the body without being metabolized or broken down." For more information or to order the product check *www.sucralose.com*. A product of McNeil Specialty Products Company, a subsidiary of Johnson & Johnson, Splenda is 3 times sweeter than NutraSweet and also contains no calories. It is already used in commercial products such as Ocean Spray brand low calorie juices. It will be sold shortly in supermarkets. Right now it can be purchased from the web site. For more information call 1–800–777–5363 or write: McNeil Specialty Products, P.O. Box 604, Dept P, Berkeley Heights, NJ 07922–0604.
- Almond milk can be ordered from Pacific Foods of Oregon, Inc. Tualatin, Oregon 97062, 503–692–9666, *www.pacificfoods.com*.

# Equipment

- A three-inch herb/tea ball (made in China) can be ordered from Progressive International Corp, Kitchen Accessories for Healthy Cooking, Kent, Washington, 98032. Imported in Canada by Par counselTron, Richmond Hill, Ontario, L4BIL2, dishwasher safe, stainless steel.

A stainless-steel mesh tea infuser, Farberware #77270, with a lifetime limited warranty, can be ordered c/o Lifetime Hoan corporation, (service dept), P. O. Box 921 Dayton, NJ 08810.

# Bibliography

*Prevention's New Foods for Healing*. Selene Yeager and the Editors of *Prevention Health Books* (Rodale Press, Inc. 1998).

*The PDR Family Guide to Natural Medicines and Healing Therapies* (Three Rivers Press, 1999).

*The Medical Advisor, The Complete Guide to Alternative and Conventional Treatments* (Time-Life Books, 1997).

*A Handbook of Natural Folk Remedies*. Elena Oumano, Ph.D. (Avon Books, 1997).

*The Natural Pharmacy*. Skye Lininger, D.C., ed. (Prima Health, 1998).

*Herbs of Choice*. Varro E. Tyler, Ph.D. (Pharmaceutical Products Press, 1994).

*The Complete Book of Ayurvedic Home Remedies*. Vasant Lad, B.A.M.S.,M.A.Sc. (Three Rivers Press, 1999).

*The American Dietetic Association's Complete Food and Nutrition Guide*. Roberta Larson Duyff, M.S.,R.D., C.F.C.S. (Chronimed Publishing, 1996).

"Communicating Food for Health." Carol M. Coughlin, R.D. (January 2000: p. 9).

"Boost Your Brainpower." Ellen Michaud, Russ Wild and the Editors of *Prevention* magazine (Rodale Press, Inc. 1991).

``Topics in Nutrition, Women, Food, and Mood." Mindy S. Kurzer, Ph.D. Hershey Foods Corporation (September 1996).

**drink to your health**

"What Is SAMe?" *Newsweek.* Geoffrey Cowley and Anne Underwood (July 5, 1999).

*True Thai.* Victor Sodsook, with Theresa Volpe Laursen and Byron Laursen (William Morrow and Company, 1995).

"Women Need to Beef Up Dietary Zinc." *Tufts University Health & Nutrition Letter* (January 2000, vol 17, No. 11: p. 1).

"Killing Bacteria—with Cinnamon?" *Tufts University Health & Nutrition Letter* (October 1999, vol 17, no. 8: p. 2).

*Baking Soda.* Vicki Lansky (The Book Peddlers, Deephaven, Minnesota, 1995).

"Food Sources of Added Sweeteners in the Diets of Americans." *Journal of the American Dietetic Association.* Joanne F. Guthrie, Ph.D., M.P.H., R.D.; Joan F. Morton, M.S. (January 2000, vol. 100, No. 1: p. 43–48).

"Water: The Elixir of Life." *Current Concepts and Perspectives in Nutrition.* Barbara Levine, Ph.D., R.D. (February 1999, vol. 9, No. 1: p. 1–8).

# Index

**drink to your health**

**drink to your health**

**drink to your health**

**drink to your health**